Praise for MICHAEL HARRIS *and*
FALLING DOWN getting UP

Michael has already shared his story with many. He tells it well and he often tells it without words. His story manifests in how he presents himself in the world - to friends, family, acquaintances and strangers. But when he does put words to his story, you cannot help but feel connected.

—**Esther Oh**, Co-Director Bikram Yoga,
Burnaby, British Columbia

The unique insights Michael has acquired will benefit many.
—**T.A. Long**, Old Friend

Whether it's strutting through the midst of 400 students to the theme of Rocky to teach a Bikram class; or sitting mellow in a small circle of 10 getting real in Acapulco, Michael is your man.
—**Wendy Crowther**, Yoga Teacher

My colleague and mentor for 11 1/2 years, Michael is one of those rare individuals who walks the walk, and talks the talk...I aspire to be like him in my own daily teachings and practices to emulate his wholeness.

—**Amy Pittelkau**, Director Bikram Yoga Fresno

Michael's one of my dearest friends. I admire how approachable he is to everyone. He can relate to all walks of life which is only a small component of how he inspires people. I'm so lucky to know him.

—**Michele Vennard**, Director/Owner Bikram Yoga San Jose

I have only known Michael as who he is today but have heard his story. I would never have known he went through all he has. What an inspiration.

—**John Herbik**, Magazine Publisher

Michael didn't just "fall down", he full on "wiped out", figuratively and literally!

—**David Groves**, Yoga Teacher

In Michael, I have found a friend who is spiritual, funny, smart, self aware, motivating, supportive, loving, open, generous, and emotionally intelligent. Everyone deserves to hear Michael's inspiring story; the experiences and choices that made him the man he is today.

—**Rachel Hayward**, Student

In a world full of new-age nonsense, Michael is a true gem. He shines with integrity, compassion and real-life wisdom. Actually walking the talk, he continues to bless us all; thank God he finally has written a book!

—**Jessica Biskind**, MA, LPC

FALLING DOWN getting UP

FALLING DOWN
getting UP

A STORY OF OVERCOMING LIFE TO LIVE

MICHAEL HARRIS
founder of The Getting Up Project

NEW YORK

FALLING DOWN getting UP
A STORY OF OVERCOMING LIFE TO LIVE

ISBN 978-1-61448-235-2 Paperback
ISBN 978-1-61448-236-9 eBook
Library of Congress Control Number: 2012931102

Morgan James Publishing
The Entrepreneurial Publisher
5 Penn Plaza, 23rd Floor,
New York City, New York 10001
(212) 655-5470 office • (516) 908-4496 fax
www.MorganJamesPublishing.com

Cover Design by:
Rachel Lopez
www.r2cdesign.com

Interior Design by:
Bonnie Bushman
bonnie@caboodlegraphics.com

In an effort to support local communities, raise awareness and funds, Morgan James Publishing donates a percentage of all book sales for the life of each book to Habitat for Humanity Peninsula and Greater Williamsburg.

Habitat for Humanity®
Peninsula and
Greater Williamsburg
Building Partner

Get involved today, visit
www.MorganJamesBuilds.com.

*This book is dedicated to
my mother and father, who
taught me much more than
I have ever admitted.*

AN OPENING THOUGHT.

It took me a while—
but I finally discovered an idea that
might be obvious to others.
This is the thought:

That as a child, when I was first learning to crawl, then learning to walk, I was falling down all the time. Without judgment, my parents would just tell me to get back up.

Then why was it that as I grew older and then became an adult I would judge and criticize myself whenever I would fall?

Perhaps falling down and getting back up
is just part of the deal.
Regardless,
as long as I continue to be alive,
I will keep getting back up.

ACKNOWLEDGMENTS

The actual creation of this book took a lifetime. The writing happened in fits and spurts over 10 years. In that time there have been many individuals who have supported my efforts, either directly or indirectly. A group of individuals who never actually saw the manuscript or directly helped in the writing of the book have been the greatest support I could have had. That group is the yoga teachers who have worked for me as the final book was being written. These teachers and friends are Eva Vidal, Susie McLagan, Delana Miller, Sherry Brooke and Anne Jackson. These outstanding individuals stepped up to teach and run the yoga studio so I could indulge myself in writing this book. I send the deepest gratitude to each of you.

There have been many others who have also guided, helped and supported my efforts. Alon Sagee has listened to me for years. Ann McIndoo gave me the kick start to begin writing again. Louise Hawker edited the final version. Steve Harrison and his associates have taught me how to believe in myself. My publisher Rick Frischman believed in me and my project.

Bikram Choudhury, my yoga teacher for so many years, taught me to step up to the plate no matter what. Rajashree Choudhury is an ongoing source of inspiration for all that I do, and Emmy Cleaves always reminds me to just get up and do it.

Over the years there have been many friends and family who have helped me in so many ways. Whether they knew it or not, these friends have given me nudges and encouragement just at the right moments. Thank you to all of you, whether I mentioned you or not.

CONTENTS

FOREWORD

By Jay Conrad Levinson

M ichael Harris would never have had the courage and wisdom he displays in this enlightening book had he not experienced a multitude of falling downs and getting ups. He has been there, done that, bought the t-shirts, and walked the walk. Here, for our benefit, he talks the talk.

Blessings should be bestowed upon him for rather than regale us with advice, he regales us with a story, one that will enthrall you in the reading as much as must have enthralled him in the telling.

I envy you because you are poised at the threshold of such a story. It begins where there really is no beginning—deep in the environs of a coma—and meanders to places that may be familiar and definitely will be fascinating to you. Your guide will be Mr. Harris, bruises and all.

What you are about to read is all the more astonishing because it emanates from the most profound teacher of all—the truth. What you learn from it is yours forever.

Rarely does an author reveal so much viscera but Mr. Harris reveals it because it is there. If he didn't you might not so ably get up after falling down.

I know you're going to appreciate the journey you're about to take, and to feel grateful to Michael for taking it before you.

—Jay Conrad Levinson
Father of Guerrilla Marketing

INTRODUCTION

Hello everyone, my name is Michael and this is my story. Frankly, the writing of this book has been more than eye opening. To reflect on my journey in life, it is hard to believe that, as my favorite comedian Steve Martin says, "I'm a wild and crazy guy."

Was it really me that was in a coma for 10 days and told by the spirits to get back to my body? Yep, it happened. Was it really I who nearly drank himself to death after having 60% of my liver removed? It just seems so absurd. Yet it happened. What seems even more absurd is that I am still alive to tell you. My story will take you from growing up as a child in Portland, Oregon to buying hashish in Morocco and to my passion for yoga. You will read many, but not all, of my stories about drinking and causing trouble.

As several doctors have said, "Michael, you are lucky to be alive; you should be dead." "Really, I should be dead? Huh, I swear I am still here." At least today I am, and for that I am grateful. I tell how I survived a near death experience to live a pretty darn good life. I'm not wealthy and I don't own a lot of stuff. Well, I can be a pack rat. What I do have is a deep gratitude that I am alive. That I have an incredible family and group of friends that I get to take this journey with. Trust me— not everything is perfect. I make plenty of mistakes. I have burned a few bridges. Ever notice how bridges are so colorful when burning?

Once I get through all the gory stuff, I tell you how I made it through. How I "walked through the pain" when the doctors told me that I would lose my legs from vascular disease. How grace and something much bigger than I am kept the light burning on the journey to a better life. You will read how I became a successful yoga teacher and a business mentor. Wherever I am in life, there always seems to be something guiding and nudging me to get out of the hell I was living in and to do something greater. Something that was pushing me on my cane to take just one more step. Something that has always kept reminding me to never give up before the miracle.

When you are done with this story, I hope that you are entertained. That is what a good book will do. Perhaps you will find the strength and the courage to look at your life and how you live. Are you living the life you want? If not, why not? No one else can do it for you —only you can live your life. To help "nudge" you on your way I have made a few simple suggestions that just might be what you need to start your own "getting up project." Thus truly living the life that only you can imagine.

CHAPTER 1

FALLING DOWN

It was the summer of 1971 and I was just 12 years old. On the 20th hole, in "sudden death," I beat Bobby Atkinson for the Nine Hole Junior Championship at Portland Golf Club. Bobby and I were friends and we played golf together many times. That day was simply my turn to win, and as champ I now had the incredible bragging rights.

After the big win our family headed down to Gearhart – a small town on the Oregon coast just north of Seaside. We would play on the beach, swim in the ocean, and dig for razor clams until exhausted. At night we would frequently go to Seaside to ride the bumper cars over and over. That summer we met Batman—Adam West—my favorite superhero. His mother had a home just down the street from our rented beach house. Batman had a pretty cute daughter who was about my age. The summer was looking good!

One night a bunch of us were on the beach having a bonfire. Just a group of kids without the parents. That could be trouble. Unknown to our parents, we were smoking some pot and having a few beers. Of course, smoking pot gave us the munchies and we stuffed ourselves with s'mores and marshmallows. Our hands became sticky and gooey from pulling the marshmallows off the sticks. We got the pot from some older kids and we snuck the beer from the house. At 12 years old I already liked the feeling of being high. After all, even when we were little kids of three or four, we loved to be spun around in a circle to get that dizzy feeling. Getting high seemed so natural.

Smacking the Beach

The next day, August 30th, we headed to Cullaby Lake to go water skiing on our friends' boat. It was Lori, her sister Carleen, Joe, my brother Steve and me. After the previous night's bash on the beach I wasn't feeling that well. My head was hurting from the pot and the beer, my stomach churning from the marshmallows and s'mores. Twelve years old and I had a hangover.

The day was cool, overcast and gray. Even though it was the last week of the summer, the lake was mostly empty and there were just one or two other boats on the water. I was a decent skier— not great, but good enough to be the occasional show-off. As the boat was going around the lake, my thinking was to demonstrate just how great a skier I was and do a beach landing. Besides, my head was throbbing from partying the night before and I just didn't want to get wet. I was beginning to move to the outside of the wake, increasing my speed. Once we got closer to the beach, I saw another boat cut right in front of our boat. To avoid a collision, Carleen thought quickly and veered sharply to the left. This increased my speed on the skis and whipped me that much closer to the beach. At about that same moment, I decided to let go of the rope.

All of a sudden, my skis were sliding across the sandy beach. I don't know how fast I was going—perhaps 30 or 35 miles per hour, perhaps a little faster. Before I knew it, there was this terrible crunching sound when the skis snapped. Smack ... I hit this big old log lying across the beach. Where was my superhero Batman when I needed him to save me? At first I just lay there in pain, unable to move. My friends and brother, not realizing how serious the accident was, began to laugh. The wind had been totally knocked out of me and my whole body was covered with this terrible horrible feeling from the gritty sand. In a minute or two after falling down, I got up and ran into the water. I had to get the scratchy itchy sand off my body as fast as I could. For what seemed like forever, I felt as if I just couldn't take a breath. Like any kid, I had had the wind knocked out of me pretty good, but nothing that felt like this. This time it seemed as if I would never stop gasping for air. My head started spinning and I thought I would pass out. Very quickly, everyone realized that it was no laughing matter—that I was really hurt.

Seeing what had happened, Carleen parked the boat at the dock. By now, everyone was getting pretty freaked out and no one knew exactly what to do. Other than some good scratches on my body and lots of pain, there were no apparent external injuries. There was no blood and nothing had punctured me.

The ski boat was left at the dock as I was put in the back seat of the red station wagon. I would crunch up writhing in pain and crying. Someone decided it was best to take me back to the house in Gearhart and find my mom. To get me to the beach house quickly, Joe drove pretty fast south on Highway 101. My dad was in Portland working at the time, and mom was playing golf with Carleen's and Lori's mom at Seaside Golf Club. Lori found my mom on the golf course; she rushed back to the house to check on me. Just to be safe and to make sure I was ok, mom immediately took me to Seaside Hospital. I don't remember ever seeing a doctor there. I just remember a receptionist, a nurse and an x-ray technician. I sat on a cold hard metal exam table, feeling intense pain increasing in my stomach and chest. They took some x-rays and didn't see any problems. The nurse told me that I would be ok and said I need not cry and complain so much. After all, they couldn't find anything wrong with me, and she said I just had a few scratches and bruises. But tears were rolling down my face and my body was really hurting.

During the night and the following morning I began throwing up blood. I looked in the toilet and thought, "Where is all this blood coming from?" I was in such terrific pain and scared to death. Standing up, it felt as if there was a knife stuck in my upper back while I tried to walk. Mom saw the blood too, and decided to cut our beach trip short and return to Portland, about a 90 minute drive.

It was now close to seven at night, and we went immediately to the Children's Clinic in Sylvan. It was after hours so the night doctor, Dr. Scott Goodnight Jr., examined me. My eyes were all yellow and looked messed up. The doctor knew that something serious was happening to me. He decided to immediately send me to Emanuel Hospital to see another doctor, Dr. Timothy Campbell. Emanuel was the same hospital where I was born in 1958.

The hospital admitted me and, the next thing I knew, I was being wheeled quickly down the hall on a gurney covered with a blanket. Looking down my body, I could see where a small lump had formed just below my rib cage. This lump was about the size of half a softball. It seemed logical at the time to ask them if they were going to "sand the bump off."

For the next ten days I remained in a coma after, I later found out, a nearly 20-hour surgery. Coma comes from the Greek word "koma", meaning "deep sleep." While in the coma a doctor, a nurse or my parents would ask me to squeeze their thumb or a finger. Sometimes I could hear them. But as hard as I tried, I just couldn't squeeze or move anything. My eyes were closed and it was totally frustrating not to move or talk. I don't think they ever knew that, at times, I was aware of them and I could hear them talk. My parents were completely devastated and were told that I was not expected to live. The water skiing accident had caused massive internal injuries. The surgeons ended up removing 60 percent of my liver and my gall bladder— and I had six cracked ribs. Pretty much the whole right side of my torso had taken the tremendous impact of smacking the beach. I have no way of knowing this for sure—but years later my brother Steve told me he remembered that, up to 1971, I was supposedly the youngest person ever to have this much of their liver removed and survive. I was told that it was a complete miracle that I lived.

During the nearly day-long surgery, I used 21 pints of blood. My blood type is "B" and, apparently, there was such a short supply of B blood in Portland that even the surgeon, Dr. Campbell, who had the same blood type, stopped and donated a pint during the surgery. Dr. Campbell later told me that much of the extended time in surgery was just trying to stop the bleeding. He said that there were literally thousands of stitches, both on the inside and the outside of my body. So many stitches they didn't even bother to count. Sitting here today, I still have multiple silver clips in my body that were used to clip certain blood vessels within my chest and abdomen.

WAKING FROM THE COMA

When I was deep in the coma, something happened to me that I have only more recently realized has had a huge impact on much of my life. There was a moment that I remember being out of my body and looking back down to see it. I could see the whole room and my body lying on my back in bed. Then all of a sudden, I was surrounded by five or six people who were in long dark robes in a garden area. There were lots of plants and trees everywhere. This place and the people there felt like a totally safe and peaceful place.

It seemed like I was at home in my surroundings. There was absolutely no pain at all in my body or mind. I felt whole and complete. These people, or what I call "spirits," were somehow there loving and protecting me. We were all talking—though I don't remember much of what was said. Just as quickly as I arrived, I suddenly felt that I was moving away from them, that I was leaving this place to go back to my body. Immense sadness began to engulf me—I didn't want to go back. I told them that I didn't want to leave. As I reached back, I begged them to let me stay. What I heard, from what seemed like the leader was, *"You are not through with your life; it is time to go back."* Huh? I looked back at them and felt great sorrow that I was leaving this place of amazing love and acceptance. I was getting told to leave the garden.

The next thing I knew I was back in my body. I could feel all the tubes—they were everywhere. Nose, mouth, penis and both arms all had tubes. Shortly thereafter, I opened my eyes and began to slowly awaken from the coma. Had I died and come back? Where were my spirit friends from the garden? I tried to pull the penis tube out because I didn't like it. A nurse saw me and came to fix it. Later I was told that the first words the nurses heard me speak were "Bike, 30 days." Hey, I was a 12 year old kid and my bike was at Kissler's Bike Shop getting repaired. Mom and dad had apparently forgotten all about my prized possession. But if I was back, I wanted my bike and I wanted it right now. After all, if I wasn't through with life yet, there were places to go and things to do!

Since my surgery, my parents had virtually camped out at the hospital. They were more than overjoyed that I had come out of the coma and was still alive and breathing. Even though I was still in pretty bad shape, they could now have increased hope that I might survive. That perhaps their prayers to God had spared their little boy's life.

While I continued to remain in ICU, my temperature began to soar. To help reduce my growing fever, the doctors put some type of cold mattress under my body. I didn't like the mattress at all, it was freezing. Then my right lung collapsed and I was struggling to breathe once again. Dr. Campbell was called to my bedside right away. Being fascinated at what he was doing, I watched him insert a small metal tube between my rib cage and into my lung. This tube was connected to a gallon size bottle by a hose. My temperature slowly began to drop and my lung had started to re-inflate. It was working and my breathing began to improve. After another day or two, Dr. Campbell took the red rubber tubes out of my arms. When he pulled them out I was amazed how long each one was. There were two tubes in each arm that had been inserted just above the inside of my elbow. Each tube seemed like at least a couple of feet long. He told me that the tubes had been inserted as close to my heart as possible.

Another one of my memories in ICU was another patient that I could see in the bed across the room. I'm not sure how old he was. I just remember him lying in a twisted position and moaning from time to time. When I asked the nurses what was wrong with him, they told me that he was an alcoholic and had cirrhosis of the liver. It was the first time that I saw a dying alcoholic. I thought that he must have come from skid row. *I don't know whether he survived and it certainly never occurred to me that one day I could be a drunk too.*

Eventually the doctor moved me to the pediatric wing of the hospital. There was a small room next to the nurse's station that had been used for storage. Dr. Campbell had everything moved out of this room and then set it up with a bed for me. It was a perfect room because it had a window in it so the nurses could always see me. In the other room next to me there was another kid that had been burned over a large part of his body. It struck me that he might not survive and die. After a couple more days he did pass away. It was somewhere around then that I began to realize that I had been very lucky and was somehow going to make it and live. *I had the memories of the spirits and the garden and felt some comfort.*

Because I was such a rare and unusual case, a lot of different doctors came to look at me. They wanted to see how this kid was still alive after such horrendous injuries. One day there was a doctor from the East coast who saw me. I think that he was from Philadelphia. He came with a whole group of doctors, including Dr. Campbell. He was examining me and looking at my chart and asking my doctor a whole bunch of questions. What stands out the most was when he said that he would have given me a tracheotomy. When they told me what that was, it gave me the creeps. I didn't like that doctor.

Being in pediatrics became kind of fun. Another kid and I had wheelchair races in the hall. We would go up and down, up and down. Most of the time I won. The nurses didn't like it much, but they were at least glad that we were both getting better. There was one special nurse who was from ICU. She would come visit me before and after her shifts and wash my hair as we talked.

GOING HOME

For the month of September, I remained recuperating in the hospital. More friends and family were now able to visit me in pediatrics. I remember receiving a lot of games as presents. Lori told me years later that the first thing she remembered when she was able to see me in the hospital, was that I was happy, that as a kid I always seemed to have a smile.

Dr. Campbell knew I could remain in the hospital for another month or two, but decided I'd be better off at home in my own surroundings. So off I went home to be in my own bedroom and with my family. Each day, the doctor would come to our house as part of his rounds. There was a still a drainage tube in the right side of my stomach for all the pus and fluids my body was producing and releasing. Each day he came he would check on me and the tube. Sometimes he would flush it out and other times he would replace it. The drain tube would remain in the side of my abdomen all the way through February. Today this scar looks as if I was stabbed and wounded by a knife. Occasionally today I will make bad jokes about getting stabbed in some nasty fight that I won.

The best part of being home was that I was around my family and my friends, and my girlfriend Laura could visit me. When I had been in the hospital, all my friends had been worried that I was going to die. Now that I was home, I was beginning to sharpen my skills playing on our nine foot Brunswick pool table. I got really good and could eventually easily sink a whole rack of balls. Now my friends were worried that I was going to win every game. My brother Steve tells me that I would play a marble game for hours, over and over again.

My parents were extremely grateful to Dr. Campbell for everything he was doing. One day they invited him to the house for dinner to honor him and tell him directly. My parents felt that he deserved much more money for "saving" me and for everything he was doing. Our family sat in our living room and dad gave the doctor a personal check. I was never sure how much that check was for. My parents had also bought a really nice watch that I got to give him directly. Dr. Campbell was always pretty adamant that he didn't save me. He said that all he really did was stitch up all the extensive damage to my organs and body. *He said it was God that saved me. I think that perhaps God saved me through Dr. Campbell's amazing skills.*

BACK TO SCHOOL

I was now 13 and headed into seventh grade and junior high. To make sure I didn't get too far behind in my school work, I had a tutor who would come to the house nearly every day. Primarily she was having me do the basic school work. Officially I didn't start seventh grade and go back to at school at Whitford Junior High until January. To get out of the house and be around my other friends at school was good, but also scary.

Most of my friends were glad to see me – though there were some kids at school who acted like total bullies to everyone and were pretty cruel. There was still the drain tube in my side and I would need go to the nurse's office each day to make sure everything was ok.

The cruelty that some kids had really surprised me. They would point and laugh at me. I was that pale, sickly looking kid that all schools have. There were various rumors floating around that I had my kidney removed or some other thing. There were many times that I tried to correct them, but eventually gave up explaining what happened. Not everyone accepted me and that hurt— a lot. But what could I do? As a result of that, today I will often support the "underdog."

Physically I was healing slowly but surely. Emotionally I was going downhill fast. I just wanted to be a regular kid like everyone else. I wasn't. I had nearly died in this horrific accident and felt that I didn't know what to do or how to relate. I desperately wanted to be like the other kids. I didn't want to be sick. I didn't want to be the last one picked on a school team in physical education. I wanted to be accepted by everyone. I wanted to do any sport I wanted. When I tried to talk to my parents, they didn't seem to be able to listen me. Perhaps they were just grateful that I was alive. Mostly they would tell me that I would be ok—but I wasn't feeling ok. I was feeling angry, resentful and abandoned. There were times that we would argue about how well I was doing. My parents were simply doing the best they could. There were many moments that I experienced where I just wanted to return to the spirits I had met in my coma. *That garden I visited was the safest place I had ever been to. Why did they send me back? Why did they abandon and not accept me?*

TURNING TO POT

At some point I realized that there were certain kids who would always accept me exactly the way I was. Those were the party kids. The ones that smoked pot, used drugs and drank. Most of them were having their own struggles and difficulties that they didn't know how to deal with. My use of pot and alcohol started slowly. Dr. Campbell had said that it was probably best to stay away from alcohol throughout my life, except maybe an occasional glass of wine when I was older. So what did I do? I started smoking pot. First it was a hit or two. I liked it on the beach before the accident and I still liked it. There was so much relief from all the inner turmoil I was experiencing. The more pot I smoked the more my restlessness seemed to calm down. Very quickly I started and needed to smoke pot nearly every day. The older kids in the neighborhood somehow always had an endless supply. I soon learned that I could buy extra pot, sell a little and have my supply for free. What could be better?

By the time summer had passed and eighth grade had started, I was getting pretty wild. My hair was strawberry blonde, wavy and long. It was now touching my shoulders. Some people would call me 'goldilocks.' I absolutely hated that name. The girls liked my hair though. Especially the wild ones.

On September 1, 1972, one year from my surgery, Dr. Campbell had me do a liver scan. He sent me to St. Vincent's Hospital in Portland for the testing. He said that they would inject me with a radioactive dye that would determine whether or not my liver had grown back. Cool, the liver grows back. As they were performing the test there was a monitor there that I could sit and watch. While watching the monitor it looked like my liver had fully grown back. Indeed that is exactly what Dr. Campbell said. They didn't know whether it had taken a few months or the whole year. They just knew that it was now grown back to full size. I guess I was lucky that one of the right organs was damaged in the accident.

Of course I was still healing and had some ongoing daily pain. I was reminded not to participate in any contact sports. Dr. Campbell said I couldn't play football because he didn't want me to get hit in the abdomen or chest. He thought it would still be too risky. I was told I could begin to play baseball again. Dad had built a baseball field in our back lot and playing ball was always one of my favorite sports. All the neighbor kids would come over and we would spend hours just trying to hit the ball as hard as we could.

My interests, though, still included smoking pot. Could that be an interest? I don't know exactly what day it was, I just know that at some point I began to think inside of me that I could drink a little. After all, my liver had grown back and maybe it was ok to drink. Maybe the good doctor was wrong.

My parents always had a well-stocked liquor cabinet. Dad would buy booze by the case and store it against the wall in the garage. I would steal some bottles now and then and share it with the neighbor kids. I started drinking more and more. I really liked the feeling of being high and drunk. Sometimes I would get sick and throw it all up, but it didn't stop me. The hose of drugs and alcohol in my life was getting turned on. I learned that when I was high I didn't need to deal with the painful emotions from my accident. If something came up, I lit a bowl of pot or drank some booze.

NOOSE MAN

In ninth grade I had a close call with the neighborhood pot dealers. One day I got off the school bus with my saxophone and they were all waiting for me. There were four of them in a van and they asked me to get in. I didn't give it a second thought and pulled out a cigarette. Yes, I had started smoking too. They said, "Don't light that." Ok, something is going on—something is wrong. We drove a few blocks to one of their houses. When we got out of the car they brought me to the side of the house where one of them had a long rope. In front of me he started making a noose. He seemed to know what he was doing with a rope. Were they going to hang me? They said, "Where's all of the pot you took? You were the only one who knows where it was hid. There's 12 pounds of pot you stole." Terrified I said, "Ahh, it wasn't me."

"We're going to put you in this noose and hang it over that tree then leave you for the Doberman pinscher." They're going to do what? I hadn't stolen any pot and I kept denying it over and over. Finally I said even though I didn't do it I would pay them for it. I was petrified they would hurt me, but eventually they let me go. I walked home with my sax and hid in the bushes in the corner of our yard. I was trembling and scared and I didn't want to go in the house—my Mom was there. After a while I calmed down enough to go in. Right away mom knew something was wrong with me. I just told her that I wasn't feeling well. I certainly wasn't feeling well and went straight into my bedroom. I was scared totally shitless. *Going back to the garden to be with the spirits sounded really good again. Yet if they kicked me out the first time, they just might do it again.*

The next day I was walking down the street from the store and one of the guys pulled up in his car. It was noose man with his girlfriend snuggled up against him. There was really no place to run and hide. He asked if I wanted a ride, then smiled. He said, "I'm really sorry Michael. We know you didn't take the pot. It turns out mom found it hidden behind the wood pile and burned it up in the fireplace." Oh, what relief— he wasn't going to hurt me after all. He then offered to make sure I could keep getting as much pot that I wanted from him. That was good because I thought that I had lost my supplier.

CHAPTER 2

WHO IS MY FAMILY?

In spite of what I have said so far, growing up in Portland was often filled with great fun and laughter. Our family had a joke about a handshake from the movie "The Bank Dick." In the movie, W.C. Fields had just foiled a bank robbery. The bank robbery occurred in January 1933. As a reward, the bank president gave W.C. Fields a 1932 calendar and a hardy handshake. The "hardy handshake" was really just a light touching of the palms and wasn't a shake at all. Our family would do this light handshake with each other and just howl laughing. Sometimes we just couldn't stop the joke.

My father was a successful oil and gas jobber. When his father died of a heart attack at 52, dad left college and took over the family business. My dad grew this small chain of gas stations into what became one of the largest oil distributors in Oregon. At one point Harvard did a study of the company and couldn't

15

determine whether it was a gas and oil business or a real estate investment company. Over the years, the great majority of the company has been sold.

My mom grew up on a farm in western Minnesota. There were seven brothers and sisters who lived in a small house near the Fargo/Moorhead area. Later, mom told me that, during the depression they had very little money, though they were never hungry. There was always plenty of food to eat that they would grow on the farm. During WWII my mom's family was relocated to Portland by the government. My grandfather and mom went to work on the docks at Swan Island as welders. She later left the docks to work in cosmetics and model at Meier and Frank's. She and Dad had their first introduction at a chance meeting while she was working as a secretary for a friend of dad's. About a year later they married.

Mom and Dad built their dream house that became our family home in 1957 on the west side of Portland. Dad had bought an extra lot and ended up building a baseball field for all the neighbor kids. That field became a neighborhood focal point for all sorts of great fun and normal kids' mischievousness. As we grew older, dad built an addition to the house that became our game room. We had plenty of room for a pool table and a ping pong table. Then there was the swimming pool. This was built as we were just going into high school. The neighborhood party house was now complete.

There were many other times of fun, laughter and play. Both Christmas Eve and Christmas Day were normally celebrated at our house. On Christmas Eve my mom's side of the family would come over. There were often 30 or 40 family members eating, joking and opening presents. On Christmas Day my dad's side of the family came over. There might be 12 or 15 people and we would have a more formal Christmas dinner in the dining room. My oldest brother Bill was a real jokester at times. It was a hoot to see him hanging a sterling silver spoon on his cheek. My brother David would have a few good quips of his own. And my brother Steve always had a good joke or two to add into the fun.

Bill started playing the clarinet in the second grade. A few years later he started the sax and eventually added the piano and flute. In addition to his several college degrees, he went on to become a successful businessman. However he will still play his sax for hours every day. Because of Bill I picked up the sax in ʰ fifth grade. Though I never became a master musician like him, I enjoy playing from time to time.

My brother David grew up and was quite diligent in school. He went to work for several companies and wherever he worked he became part of upper management very quickly. In his 30's he rejoined my father's and uncle's oil and gas businesses. David held several top positions within the various companies. Eventually he became a highly regarded and successful franchisor for taking one company from about 100 locations to several thousand locations throughout the United States and Canada. He is now retired and plays golf, practices yoga and has become a passionate and competitive ballroom dancer.

My brother Steve spent much of his earlier years in the family business. At first he would run individual locations, and later managed multiple sites. After leaving the family business Steve dedicated a number of years to helping those struggling through life. In the midst of a very busy life he became the father of four kids and two step kids. Each of these kids has now grown to develop lives of their own. Today, Steve is working in management for a restaurant company with multiple locations.

In the late 60's dad bought a rent-a-car franchise in Honolulu and an oil distributor in Hilo. As kids, we often flew back and forth to Hawaii. We would have extended vacations staying in the old cabanas at the Halekalani or a rented apartment near Diamond Head. It was a great time to be kids and playing on Waikiki Beach. We learned how to surf from Wendell and Nathan, the beach boys at the Halekalani. Many times, at the end of the day of surfing, we would go back out with the outrigger canoes, paddling hard and screaming in more fun. Of course, at that age, we had a blast chasing the girls up and down the beach in their bikinis. Much of growing up was fun and fairly normal.

DAD'S PASSING

The last time I saw my father alive was when he and my mother were headed back to their home in Palm Desert. With mom next to dad, I was pushing him in a wheelchair down the concourse of the Portland Airport. It was late March 1985. He had a heart attack in early February in Palm Desert. It was his third. They had come home to Portland to see his doctors and were ready to go back to the desert. He had his green oxygen tank with him, and I kept thinking how much I wanted him to get up and walk again. *There must be something that I could do, something to help him heal, something to help him walk.*

Dad ended up passing away way too young, of a heart attack, in Palm Desert on Mother's Day, May 12th, 1985. His diagnosis had not been good. He was suffering from congestive heart failure, atherosclerosis and diabetes. He had struggled much of his life with health issues. As a 10 year old, he had a routine operation for mastoiditis to drain an abscess. During the operation he vomited and drowned. After his heart stopped for a period of time, he was revived. When this happened he had to learn how to walk and talk again. This probably made him an even more determined man later in life.

CHAPTER 3

TURNING UP THE POT

If much of growing up was so fun and relatively normal, what happened to me? Very early in my life I essentially became totally uncontrollable—especially after the water skiing accident. It was as if that huge hose was turned on and out came this endless supply of alcohol and drugs. There was really no time in my life that I could "handle" any of it. I first experimented with alcohol and pot shortly before the water ski accident. The day of the water ski accident I had quite a headache from drinking beer and smoking pot the night before. Twelve years old and I had already hit a major bottom in my career of alcohol and drug abuse. Perhaps if I had connected the dots sooner my life would have been much different. After many years of abstinence, I realized that the water skiing event was really my first alcohol related accident.

When my physical healing was coming along, I kept feeling as if my unsettled emotions were totally tearing me up. Today I still feel like I have not realized all of my unsettled feelings from the accident. Perhaps writing this book is helping me to sort it out. When I was a kid I would go to my parents and tell them that I felt like I was healing physically, but not healing emotionally. We would argue and fight about whether or not I was ok.

There were feelings and emotions coming up that I simply did not know what to do with. I was angry and feeling that my parents had abandoned me. I developed a deep resentment towards both of them. At the same time, I was feeling deserted by the spirits for kicking me out of the garden. Why did the spirits send me back to my damaged and injured body? An even deeper resentment towards God was growing and developing. I always believed in Him. I was just pissed and had that ongoing abandoned feeling from Him too. I still did not understand my near death and out of body experience when I was in a coma. *The garden in my near death experience seemed like a much better place than being here—but was it really?*

I began to turn more and more to pot. At first it was just the few hits with the other kids. We would go behind our tool shed or into the woods to our tree forts. Very quickly smoking pot became part of my daily life. I couldn't get enough of it. We would have major smoke outs everywhere. I started buying larger quantities of pot—maybe a quarter- or half- pound. If I had enough money I would buy a little more. The best thing was that I didn't need to deal with my painful emotions and the other kids would come to me for their pot. I found that I was "accepted" by this expanding group of friends. Perhaps I was becoming the king of the neighborhood.

As my pot use kept growing, other drugs would show up too. There would be lots of hashish. Someone I knew back then was bringing it in from Turkey. To see those round disks of hashish with a Turkish government tax stamp on it was strange. There were plenty of mushrooms in Oregon. Once it was discovered that these little fungi were growing everywhere and would make us hallucinate—well, I thought that was pretty incredible. Window pane acid worked too – but mushrooms were free for the picking. Mescaline, angel dust, elephant—all sorts of different drugs started circulating that we experimented with. Just about anything to get high worked. About the only thing I never did was put a needle in my arm. Getting stuck with a needle happened enough to me in the hospital.

By fourteen, alcohol started creeping in more and more in my life. Occasionally I would have a small swig from someone else's drink. In the back of my mind I kept remembering what the doctor said, "It's not good for you to ever drink." Somehow, I must have forgotten. Remember that fire hose? The fire of emotions inside of me kept getting bigger and hotter. To compensate for all this discontent, alcohol started pouring into my body as fast as I could get it—trying to put out the fire of pain. Not only was I frequently stealing dad's booze, but I also discovered a little store in the neighborhood where they would sell me beer—at fifteen years old.

My alcohol and drug abuse kept jumping and escalating to the next level. I had become a daily user of some type of substance. Almost anything would do as long as I didn't have to feel worthless inside. I wasn't at all like the other kids. I had huge scars all over my abdomen and chest. I was scared that others would not accept me anymore. Perhaps more scared that I couldn't accept myself. I needed to prove that I was still somebody. Somebody that other people would like.

My parents were at a loss and didn't know what to do with me. I thought that I had been hiding the pot and drinking pretty well, though they began to sense and realize that I was totally out of control. Even though I was a pretty "smart kid" my grades started going downhill. I was getting report cards that had C's, D's and even a few F's. My parents would try to ground me, and I was not very willing to accept their punishment. I would just do what I wanted to do regardless of what they said. My rebel was fully in charge. Besides I wasn't going to stop using—it was "saving" me from feeling my emotions.

A NEW SCHOOL

By the time I finished junior high my parents had more than enough. They knew if they sent me to Beaverton High School my "problem" would just keep getting worse. They thought if they sent me to one of the local private schools, I would get away from the influence of other kids in the neighborhood and get better. Yeah, right. So they arranged for me to take the entrance exam at Catlin Gable—one of the best private high schools around. I'm not sure exactly what happened, but the school didn't accept me. I think my parents even tried to offer additional tuition to get me in. It didn't work.

Totally fed up, my parents took me to a children's psychologist. Maybe this guy could figure out what was going on with me, maybe not. I don't remember his name; his office was in downtown Portland. I do remember liking him from the beginning because of this funny book he wrote about life. The title was something along the lines of "Life is Like a Shit Sandwich." I could've written that myself.

The psychologist decided to test my IQ to see just how intelligent I was. I guess 149 was pretty good. Just what I had been telling my parents all along—that I was smarter than they thought. More like a smart ass who didn't care for much of anything—except alcohol, pot and an assortment of other substances.

One day my parents came home with a large black book and put it in front of me. It was filled with profiles of private high schools and college prep schools. I didn't have much choice anymore about school. I was going away somewhere and that was that. At first it was thought that I would go to a school in Idyllwild, California. It was in the hills above Palm Desert—a place where my parents had a second home for the winter. I could go to the school in the mountains and visit my parents on the weekends. We got to the point that we actually went to the school. But I had a huge resistance and didn't want to go.

Instead, I found another school I thought I would like in Steamboat Springs, Colorado. The Whiteman School was set up so that they would have classes in the morning and go skiing in the afternoon. Wow, I could do that. Besides I knew how to ski pretty well, and it was a perfect way to smoke plenty of pot. So for 10th grade I was now headed to Steamboat for school. I think that all my friends were jealous that I got to go to this incredible place. To make sure I could keep smoking, I brought a quarter pound of pot with me. That seemed like it would probably be enough to get me through until at least the Christmas break. Then I could buy more in Portland and bring it back.

The Whiteman School was small, only 59 total students. Basically split pretty close to half boys and half girls. Some of the other kids were pretty smart and wild like me. I could take the assigned classes in the morning and we would have a pot smokeout in the gondola on the way to the slopes.

In class there was a heavy focus on reading, writing, science, math and so on. At the time, Whiteman was the seventh ranked college prep school in the country—more expensive than Harvard. My school work and grades immediately shot to the top. I was getting A+ in everything. Besides if the grades weren't at a certain point, no skiing. So I made sure that I always could go skiing and could always smoke pot. There was study hall every night and I would quickly whip through whatever my assignments were. Getting the work done was easy and a piece of cake.

OFF TO SPAIN

One of the things that I liked best about The Whiteman School was that each year when the snow would begin to melt, they took the whole school—teachers and students—and head for some place warm and sunny for six weeks. That year Spain was our spring destination. The school rented an old white plantation in a town west of Marbella called San Pedro de Alcantara, part of the Costa del Sol and right on the beach. Each morning we would all get up and have tons of Spanish espresso to start the day. We would often have 10 or 12 shots each. Just another great way to have a morning buzz. After all, I didn't bring my pot with me, so I needed something to feel high.

During the morning we would have our regular classes, and we would then be able to fill our afternoon with adventure. Some days we would go play on the beach or head into the local towns on the bus. I quickly discovered that I could buy alcohol most anywhere in Spain. So every once in a while I and a few other kids would sneak a drink. I tried ouzo for the first time. Talk about totally kick butt—it is something like 96% alcohol.

A SPANISH BAR

Each week we would have the chance to take off for a three or four day journey with a teacher as a chaperon. On one of the trips, about eight of us left on the train that took a route through the beautiful Spanish countryside and several different cities. At one of the overnight spots, three of us took off into the dark of night. We ended up in a very seedy Spanish bar. Picture this—three sixteen year old American kids in a Spanish bar hidden down a dark street. We walked in, and we all felt pretty slick and hip.

The place was smoky, the lights were dim and there was a small band playing behind a sheer curtain. The three of us sat down at a round table and, before we knew it, three women came over and sat on our laps. Three hot Spanish women—we were in total heaven. One of them spoke English and asked us to buy them champagne to celebrate. Of course we would—a round for everyone. It turned out that the bar wanted to charge us about $20 US for each glass. Between the three of us we barely had $100's in our pockets. We simply did not have enough money for everyone and realized that the women were actually hookers. All three of us looked at each other, then got up and ran out of that seedy bar as fast as we could. I don't know how but we managed to get back to the hotel where we were staying. Our chaperon never knew what happened.

MOROCCO AND THE MARRAKESH EXPRESS

Another school adventure took us into Morocco. About 12 of us took the ferry across the Strait of Gibraltar from Spain to

Tangier, Morocco. Our final destination would be the city of Marrakesh. I can't tell you how many times I had heard the 1969 Crosby, Stills, Nash and Young song in my head. "Wouldn't you know we're riding on the Marrakesh Express. They're taking me to Marrakesh. All on board the train, all on board the train. All on board." Yep, we were taking the "Train to Marrakesh."

Once we got off the ferry and landed in Tangier, I realize that I was in a third world country. Before I knew it, this small Moroccan-looking man approached me in the train terminal. He started talking to me in near perfect English and said he was from Chicago. He kept asking if I knew anyone there. He seemed funny, but something was not quite right. He eventually asked if I wanted to buy some hashish. Being totally naive I said, "Of course. Can I get a couple of grams?" He laughed hysterically and said it wasn't worth his precious time. I learned quickly that in Morocco most people buy much more than a couple of grams at a time.

After some ongoing haggling between us, he reached into the hood of someone standing nearby. This guy's face was mostly shrouded by his brown robe and hood. His face was scarred and looked quite scary. He broke off a big chunk of hash and I gave him something like $10US. I thought if I bought enough of it and get it back to the States, I could make a killing selling hash back there. That never happened. Instead, what I needed first was to find a way to smoke this new found treasure trove of Moroccan hash.

Before I had a chance, someone else quickly approached me. This new guy looked much scarier than the first and appeared quite angry. He demanded that I give him the hashish I just bought. Of course I denied that I had bought anything and told him that I did not know what he was talking about. He said that only Moroccans could have hashish—not foreigners—that he would turn me in to the police if I didn't give it to him now. He said I would end up rotting in jail. He kept insisting I give him the hash and I kept denying that I had any. Eventually he took off running and I thought he was going to get the police. I threw almost all of it away, except for a small amount. We then boarded the train for Marrakesh and no one knew yet about my little illegal souvenirs.

The train to Marrakesh was like something I had only seen in the movies. The cars were made out of wood that was worn and aged enough that it looked as if it might fall apart. Going through my head, as the train went rolling down the tracks, I kept hearing the same old CSN&Y song. As I was looking out the windows, herds of wild camels were roaming around the desert.

The city of Marrakesh itself was even cooler, and we stayed in an old hotel that seemed as if it had been there forever. Our teacher/chaperon on the trip was Mr. Zaqbom. He was our history teacher and we were told he was retired from the CIA. Somehow he knew his way around Marrakesh pretty well, and he took us into the bowels of the marketplace into areas where just the locals lived. He had some friends there that joined us as we kept moving about the mysterious marketplace. At one point, we started passing a place that stank more than anyplace I had been. It was one of Morocco's famous leather factories where they cured everything in horse and camel urine.

Morocco really was a third world country. In the marketplace were scenes that I had only seen on TV back home. There were crippled people who were crawling around on their hands and feet. I saw people who would just stop and defecate right in the middle of the street. There were snake charmers who would try and grab the cobras from the back of the head. Prior to being in Morocco, I never knew that so many lived in such terrible conditions.

That night, a couple of us had dinner in a little restaurant across from the hotel. It was pretty dirty and dumpy and we were there for one reason—to try some meat that none of us had ever had. What was this mystery meat on the menu? Dog. With much curiosity and trepidation I took a bite. It pretty much tasted like any other meat, though it wasn't. Probably some wild dog that the restaurant had caught that day in the marketplace. The thought of eating dog still sends shivers up my spine.

When we got back to Spain, the police showed up at the school. This was a time when Franco was in power and the feared Federales came. They said that they knew that one of the kids—Craig—had brought drugs back from Morocco. How did they know? Craig had been on the trip, though I had no idea that he had bought anything or brought anything back. I thought it was just I that had scored hash, but I didn't bring any back. Did they know about my purchase too?

The Federales told the headmaster of the school that either Craig leaves the country immediately or the whole school had to leave. Craig was expelled from school on the spot and was out of the country within 24 hours. I was lucky that I had left Morocco without my little hashish souvenir and the police never knew.

SUMMER OF 1976

At the end of the school year I was planning on going back to the Whiteman School in the fall. I could keep getting my good grades, ski daily and be able to smoke my pot. Summer in Portland would quickly change all that. Hell on wheels would be a good way to describe my unruly behavior. I used a blue

Ford pickup that dad owned and screamed around town. The summer was filled with all the friends, the girls and the drugs I didn't have in Steamboat. It was like one long, never ending wild party. When my parents were gone, we would party all night at the house. Skinny dipping in the pool, playing ping pong and shooting pool. With our huge patio there would often be 100 or 150 kids at the house and the kegs would never run dry.

It was that summer that I tried cocaine for the first time. This was a drug that I liked from the very beginning. Line it out, snort it up. The high was amazing. The girls really liked it too. The more coke that was around, the more the girls were there too. It was expensive, so I couldn't have it all the time. Just for those special occasions. Funny how so many days became a special occasion.

MR. BEAR AND WHISKEY

In September, it was time to go back to Steamboat for school. Of course it was another one of those special occasions, so there was a big send-off party for me. Then off I went with my skis and a big bag of pot. Once I got back to school, I didn't want to stay at all. I missed all my "friends" back home and I was now back under "the rules" I didn't have over the summer. At one point, I called my parents and asked to come home. They would have none of it. I then sat down on the back porch of the school with one of my favorite teachers, Mr. Bear. He was pretty much like his name. He was a big bear. I told him that I didn't belong there, that I wanted to be at a place where I could have a glass of whiskey at the end of the day. Seventeen and I wanted a glass of whiskey whenever I wanted. He said that if I stayed I would not be able to have my whiskey. Shit, what was I going to do?

One more time I called to plead and beg my parents to let me come home. Their answer was a strong "NO." I didn't like that answer and told my parents that I was coming home anyway. I packed all my stuff up and went to a local hotel in downtown Steamboat. A couple of friends from the school came to dinner that night as we all said goodbye. The following day I bought a Greyhound bus ticket back home to Portland.

There was another kid whom I didn't know sitting on the bus next to me. Part way back he told me that he had just popped some window pane acid and was flying high. I probably would have taken some too, though, damn it, he did not have any more.

CHAPTER 4

TELEPHONE POLES
AND HOUSES

Once I returned home, I started attending Beaverton High School. This is the school my parents had tried to keep me away from in the first place. They somehow knew that I would get right back into the same crowd of partying friends. To say the least, my parents were not happy that I had left the Whiteman School and was back.

BHS seemed like total kindergarten compared to the Whiteman School. I was completely bored with the class work that was being taught. It felt easy, ridiculous and useless for anything that I would ever do. If I was so smart, why did I need to learn such stupid stuff?

That fall I was partying as much as I could. I was the party king of the school. Drinking, smoking pot and mushrooms were pretty much available and used as much as I could. Because I had totally stopped caring about anyone or myself, my grades dropped faster than a rock. Where I once was the top of my class, I was now near the bottom. I simply stopped doing my school work.

THE FIRST DUII

I ended up having three DUIIs in my drinking and partying career. My first one was December 1976. It was a fairly typical Saturday night with my party friends. Another weekend—another high school kegger.

My mom had a blue Buick Skylark with a white vinyl top. I squirreled around a lot in that car—until I wrecked it. It was about 11 o'clock and we had drunk quite a bit at the party. It was pretty common that I would easily drink 10 or 20 beers. Didn't all high school kids drink like that? A friend and I left the party and were flying down Taylors Ferry Road in the rain. As we started going downhill around a corner, the car went spinning out of control and sliding. Whack—I hit a telephone pole and knocked it right over. Oh, oh ... I was in big trouble.

Before we knew it, the police were there at the accident. A large group of people and neighbors started gathering around to see what happened. It was lucky that no one was injured in the crash. For some reason, the police did not give me a ticket that night. I must have gone into a blackout because I don't remember how I got home.

The next day the police came to the house and the officer sat down next to me at our kitchen snack bar. My parents had already been incredibly furious at me for what happened. Now this. The officer explained what had happened and asked about the other people in the car. Other people? I thought it was just one friend in the front seat. The officer said that a third person had been in the back seat. I must've been in a deep blackout the night before—I didn't know that another person was there. According to the officer, it was someone they had been looking for about some problems near Sunset High School. When he told me the name, I had no idea who it was. In front of my parents, the officer then wrote me a DUII ticket for driving drunk the night before.

When I ended up in court I was pretty nervous. What would happen to me? Was I going to juvenile detention? The judge ended up being pretty gentle on me. It was the first time that I had been caught and in legal trouble. Besides, I was still a kid. The court simply sent me to "alcohol awareness class." Movies and lectures on how bad drinking, drugs and driving were. You know the typical stuff that most kids laugh at. None of it sunk in and it didn't change a thing in my life.

THE SECOND DUII

It was May 1981 and I was about ready to get my second DUII. My parents were in their second home in the desert and I was living at the house in Raleigh Hills. That night I met up with some friends at a place in Beaverton called the Tillicum Tavern. This place had been there forever. In the late 1800's it was a stage coach stop with cabins and a brothel. There were still "ladies of the night" there—though the rooms were gone and we were now driving cars and motorcycles.

I don't know how much I drank that night. It was fairly typical to drink beer and play pool until we could barely stand. When it got near closing time, I invited about ten people over to the house to play more pool and to keep talking about some deep metaphysical bullshit. Since my parents were gone and I had the party house, it was the after-hours place to go. First, though, we needed to get some more beer to keep the party going all night long.

When I left the Tillicum, it was about 2:15 a.m. I needed to get to 7-11 before they stopped selling alcohol at 2:30. Taking the shortcut, I drove as fast as I could. Why do drunks sometimes drive with one eye closed to see better?

Suddenly, as I was driving down a straight road through the neighborhood, I found my car had hit a house. How the hell did that happen? There was no house there a minute ago. I had driven right up the lawn, over the bushes, onto the front porch with my front end against the house. Oh shit—talk about big trouble. How was I now going to get to the store and back home before my friends got there? I put the car in reverse and tried to get out. The tires just spun. I was stuck on the porch and a bush and the car wouldn't budge. Just then, the owner of the house appeared at the front door in his bathrobe in totally disbelief. Someone had just hit his house in the middle of the night. Hearing him tell his wife to call the police, I really needed to get out of there and fast. No luck, the car was firmly stuck and I wasn't going anywhere.

The Beaverton police were there before I knew it. I was totally drunk and was still trying to get the car off the porch and to 7-11 for more beer. Of course the police handcuffed and arrested me. The feel of the metal cuffs was something I never wanted to feel again. He then placed me in the back of the car for the ride to the station. How was I going to get out of this? I wasn't.

At the Beaverton Police Department they put me in a small holding cage. I still have the feeling— as if I was a penned up like a restless dog. The officer took me out, fingerprinted me, took the mug shot and processed me. Before I knew it, I was transported to the Washington County Jail in Hillsboro. Fuck, I now had my second DUII and was sitting in jail with real criminals.

I had refused to take the breathalyzer so they immediately pulled my license for 90 days. How was I going to drive now? What was I going to do? Did I really drink too much to drive? Or was I just the unlucky one that night to get caught?

Because I didn't have much money, I convinced my dad to pay for an attorney. This attorney never did do much for me. Maybe he couldn't do much for me. By the time I got to court it was January 1982 and I was quickly and easily convicted of being drunk and running into a house. The court ordered me to get an evaluation for my so called "drinking problem."

TREATMENT

My new court-appointed probation officer, Rob, sent me to an outpatient treatment center in Portland called Picard and Associates. I was pretty much a no brainer for their counselors. They said I needed treatment for alcohol. I figured I had a legal problem, not a drinking problem.

Then a weird coincidence happened. Two years earlier, in 1980, I had a roommate who had been up all night drinking with another friend. As the sun was coming up, they decided to drive to the coast. My friend's car went off the highway, hit a tree and burst into flames. Both of my friends were burnt beyond recognition. My roommate's twin brother had walked into Picard and Associates the same day and we started treatment together. We had not seen each other for some time and were totally surprised.

The courts, my probation officer and the treatment center all said that I had an alcohol problem and needed to stop drinking. The treatment center was more direct and said that I was a drunk. Really? Maybe other people, but certainly not me. Since I wasn't living on skid row I couldn't be that bad.

As part of my treatment I was required to go to outside support groups and get a court slip signed, saying I had attended. Clueless would be a good way to describe me. I found a support group that I could go to late at night that was really dark and smoky. Before I went into the meeting, I would take the tobacco out of my cigarettes and mix it with pot. As I sat in the back of the room for group, I would smoke my pot-laced cigarettes. No one ever said a thing, except "Keep coming back." Really, they wanted me to come back? They probably secretly wanted all my pot.

One day it was time for a drug test from my probation officer. For two days before that I didn't smoke any pot. Someone told me, too, that if I took a bunch of vitamins it would mask the THC in the pot. It didn't work and I was busted and in trouble.

My probation officer took me into court and told the judge to send me to jail for six months for violating the terms of my probation. Somehow I convinced my dad to pay for a top notch defense attorney to help me out of this one. When the judge, who knew the attorney, asked why he had taken such a minor probation case, the attorney said that he believed in me and that he would help me get sober. Over the objection of the DA and my PO, the judge dismissed the violation and just let me go. Nothing like a good high-priced defense attorney to get you off. But the attorney didn't do anything else and I wasn't through with my party life yet.

CHAPTER 5

DRIVING THE FOG LINE

In junior high, my grandma gave me a Nikon camera for Christmas, and photography quickly became a personal passion. Surprisingly, I was good at it right away and eventually I went to work for a national portrait company. Out of about 1,000 in-house photographers, I was almost always in the top ten in their "quality rating" system. Even in the midst of my addictions, I had a pretty good eye for a good portrait. One of the best parts of this job was traveling around to the smaller towns and cities in Oregon, Washington and Idaho.

Over the next couple of years I continued non-stop to drink and use drugs. It was not a pretty sight to see. At night I wouldn't go to sleep—I passed out. In the morning I wouldn't wake up—I would come to. Sometimes I would vow never to drink again. Then night would come and I would be back with another drink in my hand. A vicious cycle that I was powerless over became entrenched in my life.

Once again, at 25, I broke out in those cold metal handcuffs. That's the thing about drinking—you never know what will happen. In this case one more DUII. My third and, thankfully, my last arrest for drunk driving. This job as a "traveling photographer" gave me the ability to travel and drink in all sorts of hole-in-the- wall bars.

It was July, 1984 and I was headed first to Pendleton, Oregon then to Kennewick, Washington for a couple of photo shoots. In Pendleton I stayed in a little campground next to the river. My van was set up pretty cool and had a big bed in the back with lots of storage space for all my photography equipment. I stayed in the campground for four days and, every night after my shoots, I would go out to the local bars and get shit faced drunk. One day I picked up a girl who worked at the store where I was shooting and went to the drive-in theater. We didn't watch any of the movie. I was young, reckless, and trying to be a show-off photographer.

After Pendleton, I went to the Tri-Cities in eastern Washington. That day I got totally plastered drunk in some unknown bar. When night came around, I tried to find my way back to the hotel. It's pretty easy to get lost there when you're sober. The Tri-Cities area consists of Pasco, Richland, and Kennewick. It's even easier to get lost when you are drunk and you're driving. Finally, I got pulled over by the police and told them how lost I was. If they only knew how lost I really was.

Next thing I knew, I "came to" in the morning in my hotel room with an incredible hangover.. My head was pounding from whatever I had done the night before. Here I was again blacked out—alcohol induced amnesia—the previous night wiped out from my memory. The first thing I thought about was my van and my photography equipment. I had no idea where it was. It was the fourth of July and my van was not in the hotel parking lot.

I called the all of the local police and reservation police, Hanford Nuclear Plant police, not to mention county and state police. I couldn't find anyone who said they'd pulled me over. There was simply no record of any police contact with me.

Somebody finally suggested I talk to the night clerk at my hotel to see if they remembered seeing me come in. That night, I asked the clerk if she knew anything. She said, "You're really lucky. The officer brought you home from Pasco to get you back here. You were so drunk you could barely even walk." She gave me the officer's name and even though it was the Fourth of July he wasn't working that day. It took another 24 hours to reach the officer who told me where my van was parked. You'd think this would be a big warning signal for me about my drinking. It wasn't and that night I was drunk again.

SHOOTING IN IDAHO

In the meantime, I was reassigned to another photo shoot in Twin Falls, Idaho. My boss gave me two days to get over there. When I arrived on the day I was told, the local store manager where I was shooting was furious. He said, "You were supposed to be here yesterday." I called my boss on the phone and he said, "They've been screaming bloody murder, it's all your fault you weren't there." He was making me take the fall for not being there on time. So I got pissed off on the phone, left all the photography equipment and took off. But before I got off the phone I told my obnoxious boss to immediately send my final paycheck. The portrait company owed me money and I wanted it now.

What does a good drunk do in these situations? Of course I drove 50 miles south to Jackpot, Nevada, gambled and got stinking ass drunk. Losing nearly $1,000 from my pocket, I was begging the blackjack pit boss for a hotel room. It was almost all the money that I had left until my check came, and I had no place to stay. Once again I "came to" in my van somewhere on the side of the road. In my hand was the key to the hotel room the pit boss must have given me. Fuck, here we go again. I couldn't remember how I got there or what happened. Another day, another blackout.

I didn't know what to do or where to go, so I drove 130 miles north to Sun Valley, Idaho. However, I was flat broke—maybe had $50 left in my pocket. I parked my van in a little camping spot I found next to the Big Wood River. My fishing luck was dismal—I couldn't catch anything.

How was I going to eat? I was essentially a homeless drunk, living in my van next to a river and flat broke. Driving up the road I had passed a church a little ways back—the Presbyterian Church of the Big Wood. Maybe they would help me out. Feeling embarrassed, reluctant and humiliated, I knocked on the church door. The minister agreed to give me some coupons that I could use at the local Safeway for food. There was a catch—no tobacco or alcohol could be bought with the coupons. Disappoint was the word of the day. Feeling hunger pains, I accepted the generous handout and used the coupons at the store for food.

The money from my photography work would still take another week or so to arrive. I simply couldn't wait that long. So I called up my grandma and begged her for money. She was completely skeptical because I had asked her for money many times before and spent it on drinking. Regardless, she reluctantly agreed to send me some money, but it would take at least a couple of days.

I did some day labor work in town and got paid at the end of each day. Now I was digging ditches at the local hospital. What would I do at the end of the day? I bought alcohol and got drunk by myself at the little hidden campsite next to the river. The fish finally started biting so I was now able to eat something. There is nothing like fresh trout fried in golden butter on the side of the river.

Three or four more days passed and $400 from my Grandma arrived for me general delivery at the local post office. Finally, a little more money. Waiting a few more days, my final photography pay of $1,100 arrived. Now I was rolling in the dough. What did I do? Of course I got shit-faced drunk and passed out in my van on a side street in the middle of Ketchum, Idaho.

THE FOG LINE

It was a very hot day in early August and it was time to get back to Portland. Both my van windows were open and the hot summer air was blowing through as I drove down the highway. Nursing a mean hangover from the night before, I drove about six hours and stopped in Pendleton for a sandwich. First thing I did was to call my girlfriend in Portland. She did not know everything that happened and she was just excited I would be back soon.

Sitting and driving for so long got me hungry and thirsty, so I needed to eat lunch. Right in downtown Pendleton there is a little place called the Rainbow Cafe. I had been there many times before and it sounded like a perfect place to eat. Ah, a sandwich and a beer on a hot day. What could be better? That is practically my last memory of what happened that day. I must have been drinking for the next eight or nine hours around town. I vaguely remembered getting kicked out of a least one bar for being falling down drunk. I'm sure it was the same story of all my other blackouts. Drank way too much and made a fool of myself.

When I did start to drive home it was about 11 at night and I hit the pedal to the metal. My girlfriend had been waiting for hours and must have wondered where the hell I was. Damn, she is going to be one pissed off lady. I'd driven about 30 miles and was coming up to the Umatilla Army Depot. This is a place where nerve gas was stored from WWII in miles and miles of big round bunkers. Most of the time that night I was driving 90 to 100 mph. I needed to get home and I-84 is a long, straight, clear open highway. Especially late at night, there is virtually no one out there. Just maybe a few jackrabbits and some rolling tumbleweed.

That August night was different. There was one lone Oregon State trooper and me. I was driving westbound and he was headed eastbound. As I flew past him, I saw him several miles back in my rear view mirror getting off at the last exit. Hmm, he must be going somewhere on a call. Then I noticed him starting to head back in my direction with his lights on.

As he was catching up with me, I slowed down to about 85. He kept getting closer and I thought, "He's driving very fast, I wonder where he's going?" So I slowed down to 80 and moved over to drive along the white fog line on the shoulder of the highway. Get this—as delusional as I was, my left arm was out the window and I was trying to wave this cop past me. After all, something really serious must be going on ahead of us and he couldn't get by me. This kept going on for several miles. Once I realized he wanted me to stop I slowed down and pulled the van over. Gosh, maybe the nerve gas was leaking from the storage bunkers and he was trying to save me from inhaling the old gas. When he approached the van, I opened up the driver's door and fell down flat on the pavement—drunk.

Here it comes again. Next thing I knew I was breaking out in those nasty handcuffs. There was that cold metal feeling tight against my wrist. I was totally baffled that I was getting arrested for my third DUII. All I remember was having a sandwich and a beer in Pendleton. At least that's all that I could remember at midnight on the side of a lonely desert highway where I was possibly breathing leaking nerve gas from WWII.

Blackouts—alcohol induced amnesia—can do funny things to the mind. Especially to my twisted mind. The officer later told me it took eight miles to pull me over. I ended up with two tickets. He first clocked me speeding in Umatilla County and put that on the first ticket. Then he pulled me over in Morrow County and gave me the DUII. Looks as if I was about ready to have more legal problems.

The officer took me to the little OSP station office in Irrigon. After processing me, he drove me back to Pendleton to house me in the Umatilla County Jail. The place seemed very dark and I quickly passed out on the metal bunk bend. The next morning the jailers woke me up. The Morrow County Sheriff himself was there to drive me back to Irrigon for my arraignment. In his red plaid shirt, he looked like a really nice county sheriff. This time he loosely put the cuffs on in front of me and placed me in the back of his cruiser for the ride to Irrigon.

The sheriff had all my processing information and noticed the address where I was living in Portland. This was my parents' house and where I grew up. The sheriff said, "Is that the house on the corner? The long, gray house with the circular driveway?" Wow, this guy's good. I was completely blown away. I said, "How do you know where that is?" He went on to tell me that in the early sixties he had been a milkman and delivered milk to our house.

The arraignment went smoothly and they released me on my own personal recognizance. There was a catch—I could not drive for 12 hours from my arrest time. That meant I had three or four hours to kill. My van was still out sitting on the freeway, which was about 10 miles away from the little courthouse.

I started walking in the hot August sun. Another state trooper who had been at the court building picked me up and gave me a ride back to my van. He said, "I'm going to be doing some radar work near here, but you have a couple of hours before you can leave. If you drive before then, I'll arrest you." Well, ok, I guess I'm not going anywhere. Lying down in the back of the van gave me a while to contemplate my new predicament. All that I could think was, "This is crazy, why me? Do I really need to stop drinking?"

It wasn't until a year later that I went back to face the judge in that little courthouse in Irrigon. Of course I pleaded innocent. There was no way I was drunk after a sandwich and a beer. Driving for so long from Idaho on a hot summer day must have made me tired and groggy. Well, the jury in eastern Oregon was made up of farmers and their wives, and I was this city slicker kid from Portland. The officer's testimony was pretty straight forward. He had pulled over a speeding drunk driving down the white fog line of I-84 in the dark of night. Innocent my ass. The trial was over in half an hour and the jury deliberated for about 13 minutes. I was guilty, of course, and they convicted me.

Because I lived in Portland, the judge let me deal with my court requirements there. She assigned me to do four three-day weekends in jail, suspended my license for three years, pay a $682 fine and to get an evaluation to determine whether I had a drinking problem. Something was wrong here. I didn't have a drinking problem, I had another legal problem.

CONNING THE EVALUATOR

When I had the court ordered evaluation, I knew just what to say and do. There is this questionnaire to determine whether or not you have a drinking problem or might be an alcoholic. The courts often use this test to determine the level of treatment that you might require. Questions like, "Do you ever feel bad about your drinking?" or "Have you ever been arrested for drunk driving?" After my third DUII arrest and years of drinking, I was already familiar with these questions. Somehow, I conned the sympathetic evaluator into believing that I wasn't an alcoholic and had "just got caught" a couple of times drinking. Instead of her assigning me to a treatment program, she put me in an "alcohol awareness program." So I went to this program and they suggested I go to support groups for alcoholics. Been there, done that, got the t-shirt and don't want to go back.

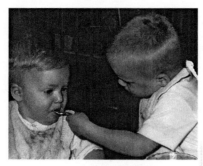

My brother Steve
feeding me. 1959

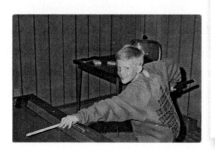

Michael playing pool. Approx 1969

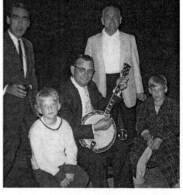

My dad's 40th
birthday party. 1966

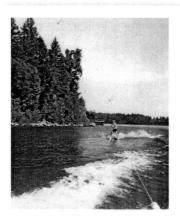

Michael water skiing before
the accident. , 1971

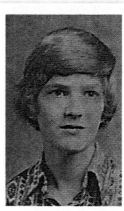

Michael, 1972, in 8th
grade one year after
the water skiing
accident.

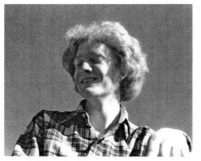

Michael, high in high school.

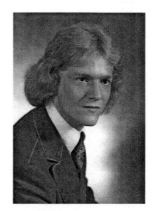

Michael's high school
senior photo.

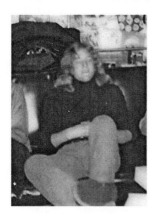

Michael, looking high
with long hair.

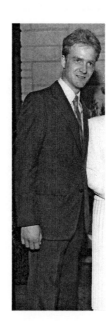

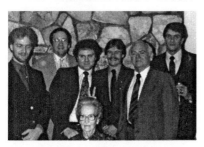

Michael (far left) with
brothers, father, uncle
and grandmother in
approximately 1980.

Michael, 30 pounds
underweight and barely
standing, shortly before
vascular surgery in 1986.

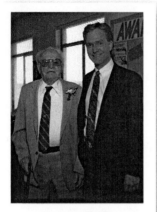

Michael with
Grandpa Lee in
approximately 1991.

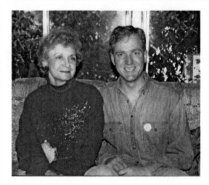

Michael with mom, Christmas
1992. (mother with cancer)

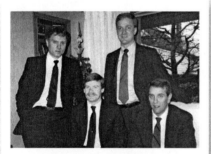

Michael with brothers
Bill, Steve and David,
approximately 1993.

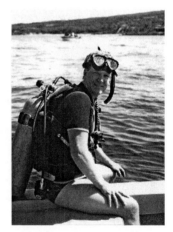

Michael diving off Maui
in 2002.

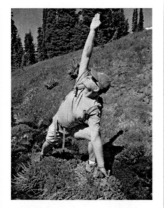

Michael in triangle in the Three Sisters Wilderness.

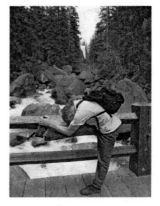

Michael in Yosemite.

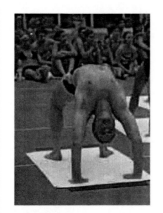

Michael demonstrating wheel pose in Acapulco.

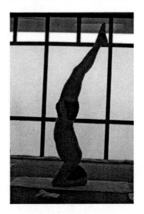

Michael demonstrating headstand.

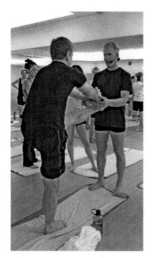

Michael leading
a workshop in
Richmond, BC.

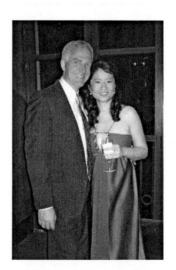

Michael with world
famous pianist Mayron
Tsong at Carnegie Hall.

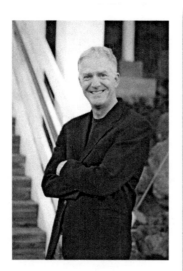

Michael today in
Bend, Oregon

CHAPTER 6

LOSING THE FLOW

On Mother's Day, May 12, 1985, my father passed away from a heart attack in Palm Desert. He was only 59, yet it was his fourth heart attack, the second in four months. It was about 10 in the morning and mom had gone out for a twenty-minute walk. When mom was out walking, dad answered a phone call from one of mom's friends. When mom returned, she found dad lying on the kitchen floor after a heart attack. He had just written a phone message for her. Seeing dad on the floor, mom grabbed a neighbor, a retired general, and called 911. All efforts to revive him failed and dad was gone.

On the day dad passed, I was working at a small photo shop in Portland. Standing behind the counter, I saw my dad's brother Dick, my uncle, walk into the store. He had never done that before and I immediately knew something was wrong. He told me what happened and I began to cry. It was a very difficult moment and I left the store for the day. The last time that I had talked to dad was about a week earlier and we had an argument on the phone about money. For so long I wished that I could've changed that.

TINGLING LEGS

Within a year of dad's death, I started getting tingling sensations in my right leg. At first I didn't give it much thought. There was some numbness, and the tingling, the kind you feel when your foot falls asleep. But over time the sensations kept getting worse, to the point where I started limping. Because I was still thinking about the next drink, I didn't seem to care much about it. I just figured whatever it was would just go away.

When a friend suggested that my spine might be out of whack I went to a chiropractor. The chiropractor examined me and she said that I didn't have any spinal problems, that it looked like I was having vascular problems. What? Here was this chiropractor that was Mayan and came from a long line of healers. I thought for sure if someone could help me, she could. I wanted her to heal whatever was going on with me. Instead, she suggested I see a doctor who specialized in vascular issues, that perhaps I could find a doctor at Oregon Health Sciences University. I didn't even have health insurance. How would I pay for that?

When I did make it to OHSU, the first doctor I was evaluated by referred me to the vascular department. The next available appointment to get in was several weeks away. On one side that was a relief, and on the other side I just wanted to find out what was happening.

Even before I had seen the chiropractor I had started walking with a cane—my dad's old brown wooden cane. At least I didn't have to pay for that. It was very difficult to walk without a great deal of pain in my right leg. At the time I didn't know it, but later the doctors told me I had intermittent claudication, a condition where there is reduced blood flow in the arteries of the leg. Incidentally, the word "claudication" comes from the Latin meaning "to limp." Limping I was good at. Limping on my leg and limping through life was what I knew. The calf would cramp up pretty good from lack of oxygen and I would have to stop and rest every 10 or 20 feet.

By the time I did get to the vascular department it was October 26, 1986. They scheduled me for a Doppler examination on both my legs. The nurse spread all this goo on my right leg that was like Vaseline. Part of their plan was to test and check both legs. That didn't make sense to me since it was just the right leg that was hurting. Part way into the examination, the nurse stopped the test and called in one of the doctors. Huh, what's going on here?

The doctor and the nurse talked about the testing so far. The doctor came over to me and looked at my right leg and foot, which was all discolored red and purple. I was told, "There are blockages in your arteries of your leg, and at this point we don't know why. We need to do further tests and an angiogram." "An angio what?" I didn't know what that was. Then he added, "We might have to amputate your right foot." I wasn't prepared for that and said the first thing that came to mind. "Fuck you, you're not taking my foot." The doctor added, "We need to check you into the hospital immediately." No way dude, I'm just too busy. I thought I needed to go do something, anything.

After my accident as a kid, the last thing I wanted was some kind of disease and a bunch of doctors cutting me open. What I really needed was a drink and to smoke some pot. I couldn't believe what was happening. How could I, at 27 years old, have vascular problems? Wasn't I an immortal man? Wasn't that some kind of old age disease? Dad died at 59. Was this related?

Four days later on October 30, I came back to the hospital and was admitted for the angio. Further testing showed my right let was 100% blocked, my left leg 65% blocked. All the blood panels were in the "normal" range. Cholesterol, both HDL and LDL, were fine. Homocystine and the other markers looked good too. So what was causing the blockages? They thought it might have been popliteal artery entrapment. This is where the muscles in the leg are pinching the arteries and reducing the blood flow. What was really going on was much more serious.

The whole vascular department was now getting involved. Dr. Porter, Professor of Vascular Surgery, and Dr. Taylor, Assistant Professor of Vascular Surgery, had taken over. My case was apparently quite unusual—27 years old and I had hardening of the arteries. They reviewed all the tests and were not able to determine the exact underlying cause. I was told that, at some point, it was likely that I would lose all or parts of both legs through amputation. Amputation? No fucking way was that going to happen. Regardless, they wanted to immediately restore my blood flow with bypass surgery on both legs. What they call a fem-pop. This is where a section of the femoral artery is removed and used to bypass the blockage in the popliteal artery. Ouch, how was I going to get through this? How was I going to pay for it without insurance? Was my drinking and smoking really affecting me that much?

LAUGHING AND SURGERY

Once all my options were explained to me, a surgery was scheduled. Not that the options were very pretty. There were some definite moments, though, of comic relief leading up to the big moment. Early in the morning of my first surgery on the right leg, some guy came into my room holding a razor. He said, "Hi, I'm here to shave you, everything from the nipples down." You're going to shave where? No one told me about this. Ok, I guess I have no other choice.

A little later that morning, before the surgery, a friend of mine who's a minister, came to my hospital room with a roll of masking tape and a pen. He said, "Let's do something. Let's write messages on the tape and put them on your legs." Besides being a minister, Haven was also a clown. We wrote funny comments on the tape like "Cut here," "Do not cut here," "Save the jewels," and so on. Laughing hilariously, we then put the taped messages on my legs. Haven reminded me that even going to surgery, even facing amputation, to always laugh and to trust in God and the universe. Both Haven and his wife Mary, also a minister, showed amazing love and support throughout the ordeal and the coming year.

Before heading to the surgical suite they started me out on some valium for relaxation. Haven had also given me a red clown's nose to wear going into surgery. Arriving in the surgical suite I was getting groggy, but I can remember when one of the doctors lifted my gown and saw the messages on my legs. The first doctor called over the other doctors and nurses and everyone there broke out laughing. If they were going to amputate my legs I, too, was going to be laughing at the absurdity of it all. Several hours later I woke in SICU and reached out for my legs. Thank God they were still there.

Three days after the first surgery they did the second fempop bypass surgery. This time it was my left leg. The prayers had been strong and endless. God, please save my legs. God, please help me. God I will do anything if you will just help me. Bargaining with God. I heard that bargaining didn't work, but it was damn worth the try. Haven and I prayed together even more. The funny messages and the red clown's nose—if it worked the first time, maybe it would work again.

This time, after surgery, I woke up delirious before they got me to SICU. There was a nurse standing over me telling me I was in surgical recovery. Inside of me there was a tremendous feeling of horrible dread. The thought occurred that I had been drunk driving and that I had injured myself in the accident. Talking to the nurse I apologized that I had killed two people in the accident. It took some time for her to convince me that it wasn't true—that I wasn't in an accident and no one died. She had to explain all about the blockages in my legs and the bypass surgery I just had. Eventually, as my mind cleared, I believed her. What was it though that caused thoughts of a drinking accident? Perhaps my fears were so great from my previous drinking and driving that underneath it all I was scared that it could actually happen.

During the second surgery on the left leg, they were able to pull out the part of the popliteal artery where the blockage was. When the artery was examined, the doctors determined that there was plaque from atherosclerosis that had caused the blockage. They now had a name for my disease. Atherosclerosis. Hmm ... my body manifesting a disease normally found in much older people. Still there was no clear determination of the Over the next six weeks everything seemed pretty smooth with my healing. Then on December 12th I was back in the hospital. I had gone in for my weekly follow-up exam. The examination showed a number of superficial thrombosis in both legs—blood clots. The doctors admitted me immediately. Shit, back in the hospital again. Now what? For the next week the doctors had me flat on my back on blood thinners.

Since the surgeries I had been feeling pretty good. The surgeries helped restore the blood flow and I was much better than ever. I would go out on the town and dance as much as I could. I was extremely grateful that I had my legs. Perhaps all the drinking, smoking and dancing since the operations wasn't really helping me to heal. Is this the reason for my blood clots? Still delusional, still in my addictions.

CHAPTER 7

GIVING UP

Once I left the hospital from the blood clots, my drinking continued to get much worse. I was so out of it my mother was no longer willing to help me or allow me to live at her house. This didn't make my mother a bad person. She was just unable to support my ongoing wild lifestyle. She was fed up and I was angry and pissed. I had just had my surgeries and had nowhere to go. I turned to a friend who reluctantly gave me a bed to sleep in. It was lucky my friend lived near a bus line. My license was still suspended from the last DUII.

On New Year's Eve 1987, I found myself at Huber's in downtown Portland. Huber's calls itself the oldest restaurant in town. I didn't care how old it was—I was there to drink 151 Spanish coffees. Making the 151's was always quite a show. Carlos would come to the table and mix the drinks up right in front of you. Of course, I always asked for just a little extra 151.

61

The last thing I remember it was about 10 p.m. and I was sitting in a booth with a few other people. I have no idea who they were. The next thing I knew I "came to" fully dressed in a hotel room with an unknown blonde woman. I had no idea who she was or where she came from. Once again the night was blacked out.

What city I was in? Looking out the hotel window, it certainly didn't look like Portland. The woman convinced me that, indeed, it was Portland and that we were at the Benson Hotel on Broadway. Apparently in my alcohol induced amnesia we had hit it off at Huber's and continued the New Year's celebration into the wee hours of the night.

When I made it back to my friend's house, I smelled as if I drank all night. I had. She was pretty upset and wanted me out of her house immediately. She felt I was not a very good example to her 16 year old son. Not much I could say about that. So I packed up the only suitcase I had and stood in front of the house waiting for the bus and talking to her son. He started to say that at least I had my health. Then he stopped and said, "I guess you don't even have that." Ouch, ouch, that hurt. He was right. I had virtually nothing and I was heading to places unknown. Where do I go from here?

A few minutes later the bus came and I stepped aboard with my suitcase and my cane. Where was I going to get off? The bus was traveling down Barbur Boulevard; I rang the bell and stepped with uncertainty onto the street. There was a dive motel right there called The Portland Rose. With nearly my last bit of money I rented a room for a week. Maybe that would give me time to figure out what the hell to do. Across the street was a 7-11 store—a perfect place to get a little food and a gallon of Gallo wine.

For the next couple of days I hid out at this little motel. One gallon of wine wasn't enough, so I bought another bottle and then another bottle. I don't know where it came from but, with the bottle between my legs, I started reading a small book called "Courage to Change." This book is a collection of stories of how mostly famous people had overcome addictions and adversity in their life. I found myself reading that book over and over while drinking my wine. Perhaps if these people could do it, so could I. Anything was better than reading the Gideon Bible in the bedside table.

ENTERING TREATMENT

A moment came over me and I decided I had enough of my crazy life and needed help. If I could somehow get to a treatment center, maybe they could help turn my life around. In reality, I also wanted a roof over my head and a safe place to sleep. I finally convinced a rehab center to let me in on my word that I would pay sometime in the future. I told them that I had about $10,000 in stock that I could sell and pay for the treatment. I really didn't.

Then I called one of my drinking buddies and told him that I had had enough, that I was done drinking. Being one of my drinking companions, he agreed I needed to stop. With a couple packs of cigarettes in my pocket and the book "Courage to Change," he drove me to the inpatient treatment center. It was January 7, 1987.

Drinking had totally defeated me. Just a year or so after having more than half my liver removed in 1971, at 13 years old, I started serious drinking. Now, just 16 years later in 1987, my body was dying from vascular disease and I was broke. I was still using dad's old brown wooden cane to walk. At this moment

I was no longer able to function like a normal person in society. Insanity had taken over. I couldn't think straight. My family had rejected me. Much of my life had been a blackout. I was chasing the drink and the drugs so I didn't have to feel my feelings. I ended up in a dive motel next to one of my dad's old gas stations. I was experiencing incomprehensible demoralization. Alcohol had taken over and I was a drunk. The only shred of hope I had was from the stories in the little book from the motel.

Checking in at the treatment center wasn't easy. I was living a lie that I could even pay for my stay. Either I was a good con or they could see right through me and wanted to help. Because of my total lack of physical health, they acquired my medical records. Several conditions were put on my admission to the program. I had to commit to follow everything they told me to do. Eat when they told me. Go to group when they told me. Sleep when they told me. Well, ok, at least I had a bed and some food. They searched my bag to make sure I didn't have any drugs or alcohol. I didn't. The final condition was that I had to quit smoking immediately. Really, I had to? They told me that it was affecting my health to such an extreme that it was part of my addiction. *So at that moment I let it all go. Alcohol, drugs and cigarettes. All substances, all at once. If I wanted to live, there was no other choice.*

When I started treatment I would hear all sorts of other people's stories. Several times a day all the patients would have group. We would sit in a big circle and share what was going on with us. Some people started talking about living on the streets, some would talk about prison, some would talk about fighting, some would talk about no money, and some would talk about suicide. Some of it I could relate to, some not at all. I had been to jail, though never prison. I'm thankful that never happened.

Many people would talk about killing themselves. How their behavior and drinking caused thoughts of not wanting to live. I never had any suicide thoughts. I always wanted to live. I always wanted to celebrate something one more time.

Throughout my drinking career I was a "happy drunk." I liked to party and celebrate. It didn't matter what it was that was being celebrated. It could've been anything. Maybe it was some type of wedding. Maybe it was a new job. Or perhaps it was simply Tuesday. It didn't matter, any reason would do. Anything to live it up. I rarely drank alone, except I might have had a drink prior to going out drinking. I rarely drank in the morning, unless I had been up all night. I would have my own all-night parties or go out on the town. Again, it didn't matter. If I was going skiing on Mt. Hood, I would bring a bota bag of wine, some pot and a pipe. Virtually all my activities required alcohol as a starter. It was the only way that I knew how to live. If there was no alcohol, there was no party.

As the days in treatment continued, the patients would begin to open up more and more. A lot of patients were really angry. More than once fights or near fights had to be stopped. The tears on my own face began to fall. Without the alcohol or drugs, the flood of emotions started. I had begun to sense that I had a huge pile of resentments, anger and emotions that I had never learned to deal with or process. Now here I was learning a new way of life. That it was my own thinking that got me into the mess I was in. That there was no way that my thinking was going to get me out.

It was suggested that I needed to find a power greater than myself. I had always believed that there was a God. As a child I had been baptized Presbyterian and went to Sunday school and I had met spirit beings in my coma. But when had God ever helped me? If God was such a great thing, how had I ended up here? It hadn't occurred to me yet that the reason I ended up in treatment was because of God. That once again I had been thrown a life preserver. Now I just needed to reach out to be saved.

The treatment center was based on spiritual principles. From past attempts at sobriety, I already knew what that meant. Not all of these principles seemed pertinent to me. Especially the one that suggested a power greater than I would return me to sanity. Even with my reluctance, though, I was willing to give it a shot.

Several times I met with the hospital minister and, from the first moment I met him, I thought that he was pretty cool. He had been sober for a number of years and he really listened to me. I was able to talk to him about my understanding and lack of understanding of God. I told him that I always thought God was there—I just didn't always like what He did. I told him how, as a young kid, the church would come and ask my parents for money and how that had always bothered me. I told him how I was angry at God and the spirits from my coma, because they sent me back to my body. Whatever I told him was ok and none of it would go into my treatment chart.

A week or so into treatment, I started to talk to a cute woman who was also in rehab. She had entered treatment a few days before I did. It started out "innocently" enough between us, but, before I knew it, there was something else to celebrate. My "feelings" began to emerge as we went into the chapel and made out. The staff quickly got on to our additional rehab activities. We were both confronted and accused of having sex. Wait a minute, we never had sex, we just kissed. Having sex was grounds for being kicked out. In the end we didn't get kicked out though we were prohibited from being alone anywhere together, including the chapel.

More group, more meals and a few movies on the weekend. Each week the treatment center would bring in past clients to come and tell their story. These were individuals who were now working on having a happy sober life. People who had the courage to change. These individuals were there to share their experience, strength and hope. They told their stories of how they were able to let go of alcohol and be a productive member of society. Every one of them said that it was a power greater than them that got them sober. This got my attention. If God had helped them, maybe, just maybe, God would help me. Hmm, I don't know, I was still pretty upset with God for getting me in this mess in the first place.

PLAN OF ACTION

When it was time to leave treatment, I sat down with my treatment counselor. He had a "plan of action" that we talked about for beginning to live in the world without alcohol and drugs. Much of the plan was designed for relapse prevention. Essentially what I needed to do was to never drink again, one day at a time. The basics included going to ongoing support groups, finding a new circle of friends and getting a job. The one suggestion I didn't like was to stay away from women for at least a year—especially the one from treatment. They said it could divert my attention from establishing a life of sobriety. Of course I believed that having a woman might actually help my sobriety.

Now that I had gone through treatment, mom agreed to help me financially. She gave me enough money for a small one bedroom apartment that was near the hospital and a grocery store. I wouldn't have my driver's license back for another seven months and could walk or take the bus. Actually, I could still only walk just a block or two. I still needed the cane from time to time.

Just as the treatment center suggested, I started with my "plan of action." Of course, not all the plan was followed to the "T." The woman from treatment had gotten out of rehab about a week before me. We made plans to meet at my apartment the day I got out. As soon as she got to my apartment, we had great mind blowing sex. Wow, sobriety was looking up!

Less than a block from my house was a 7-11 store, and sometimes I would go there to pick up a few things to eat. Before I knew it, Dan, the owner, had hired me to work the counter part-time. Another piece of the plan of action was in place. At first I didn't want any of my friends to know that I worked there. What would they think of Michael Harris working the counter at 7-11? Within a couple of weeks the store manager had quit, and Dan offered me the job of running the store. I took the job and was now the manager of a 7-11 store. Quickly, I learned how to run a small store and Dan had me participate in the management training at Southland Corp., the owners of 7-11. I excelled in my job, Southland liked me, and Dan would go play golf.

MORE VASCULAR DISEASE

In June 1987 I went to OHSU for a follow-up appointment with the vascular department. When the exam started, they found that my left leg had a new blockage. No wonder I was still limping. Once again, I was immediately admitted to the hospital. The newly formed blockage was at the site where the artery had been grafted. They now wanted to do another surgery, another bypass. The surgeons wanted to cut open my left leg one more time. Hearing all this really sucked. Going under the knife again was not appealing. It simply scared me.

The doctors couldn't give me any reason for my ongoing disease. They would mention several different possibilities, though nothing definitive. Having surgery every eight months was not very appealing to me. They started explaining how it was likely that I would eventually lose my legs through amputation. The statistics pretty much suggested I would be dead within 10 years.

They told me that if I didn't have surgery for the new blockage my leg would atrophy and would likely need to be amputated within six months. Really? Not very pleasant options. There just had to be a different answer than what I was hearing. I told the doctors that my mom had mentioned a place called the Pritikin Longevity Center, that they had a lot of success with diet and exercise. The surgeons said since my disease was progressing so quickly Pritikin was a waste of time.

Lying in that hospital bed, I had a great deal of resistance to more surgery. On one hand, the surgeons were some of the best in the world and more surgery made a great deal of since. On the other hand, not having an underlying cause that they could find was discouraging.

Maybe the problem was just from years of addiction to alcohol, drugs and smoking. The doctors did not like it that I told them that I did not want another surgery, that I was saying no. A few more doctors showed up. There were now eight doctors surrounding my bed telling me that I needed the surgery or I would lose my legs. Once again I said no. Somehow they convinced me to spend the night there and they would talk to me again in the morning.

The next morning they were all at my bedside giving me more reasons why I needed the surgery. They went on and on, explaining why I would lose my leg without the bypass. Something told me to say no. I don't know what it was—but I said NO. All they could do is shrug their shoulders and say ok. Before leaving they asked me to sign some AMA papers. That I was refusing the surgery and leaving the hospital "against medical advice." I signed, got dressed and was wheeled to the front door. With my old brown wooden cane I stood up and walked outside, not knowing what would happen next.

Each day, I kept walking as much as I could. This seemed to help at times, but I was still limping. Then, in August 1987, I finally had my license back. Driving would most definitely change things. I could now get to places much easier. All this driving, though, cut back on all the walking that I needed for my legs.

PRITIKIN LONGEVITY CENTER

In September, with the help of mom, I ended up going to the Pritikin Longevity Center. When I first arrived there I could barely walk. With the wall of the brick building on my left side and holding my mom's arm on the right side, we walked to the corner of the building and looked towards the beach. Pritikin was at the end of Pico at Ocean Boulevard in Santa Monica, right on the boardwalk.

The doctors at Pritikin reviewed my medical records and gave me an examination. Their approach to healing was different. Most of what they suggested was to begin a nearly vegan diet and walk as much as I could. They explained to me how "walking through the pain" would trigger the healing process. That as I walked into the pain, my leg would send signals to my brain that it was not getting enough blood. The brain would then send signals back to my leg and begin the process of building collateral blood vessels. Ok, let's give it a shot.

They made the food and I walked as much as I could. The first couple of days I was on a treadmill walking at .6 miles per hour for about two or three minutes, until I could barely stand the pain. I would stop, rest and start again. Each day I would be able to go a little bit longer. The food they made was actually pretty good. Because I was nearly 30 pounds underweight, they told me that I could eat as much as I wanted. That was good!

On about the third or fourth day, it was suggested that I begin to walk outside on the boardwalk. To get some fresh air and be by the beach sounded perfect to me. The boardwalk was flat, and there was a small wall along the path that I could sit on whenever I needed to stop. My progress continued slow and steady. As each day passed I began to walk a little more. I made sure that I was always walking tall along the boardwalk. After all there were a lot of women on roller blades and in bikinis, and the last thing that I wanted to look like was the 90 pound weakling on the beach.

My first yoga class was in the basement at Pritikin. Since most people there were really out of shape, the class was pretty simple. At the time, I didn't know or understand how yoga would eventually become such a big part of my life. My mom had done a little yoga and belly dancing when I was younger and I remember her teacher Fariba was a little crazy. Yoga just seemed like pretty weird stuff. Dad used to sit his hips on the floor between his feet and watch TV. Certainly none of us knew that it was a type of yoga posture. There was no awareness at all by any of us that hatha yoga had such tremendous healing powers.

There was an assortment of people staying at Pritikin. Some had heart disease, some had diabetes, some were overweight. Most were much older than I. At 29, I was by far the youngest one there. Besides the food and walking I did, they had a gentle yoga class. It was ok and a little easy stretching felt good.

Listening to everything they told me to do, within two weeks I could walk several miles. *This is critical - let me say that again. Within two weeks I went from walking 10 feet with the help of a wall and my mom's arm to walking from the Santa Monica Pier to the end of Venice Beach and back again.* Holy shit, I was getting better very quickly and it looked like no more scalpels would be cutting my legs.

Returning to Portland, a job offer was waiting for me. My experience running the 7-11 store and the Southland management program taught me a lot about small business and franchises. Many of the other local store owners became friends. One of the newest vendors for 7-11, Food Services of America, wanted to hire me to manage their new business in the Portland area. I accepted and ended up organizing and managing the sales account for roughly 90 franchised 7-11 stores. I was sober, my legs were better and now had a great job.

MY LAST DRUNK

For 23 months after treatment I remained free of alcohol and drugs. Nothing—not even cigarettes. I was attending support groups on a regular basis and making friends with other sober people. Slowly, I began to trust that my higher power was somehow helping me out. The guidance at the Pritikin Center kept me from more surgery and perhaps a life raft had been sent to bring me back to reality. Then there was the woman from treatment. We would argue, not see each other for a few days or a week, then make up and be back together. My friends and family didn't like her. The treatment center said stay away. I didn't.

On December 12th, 1988 I got in an argument on the phone with her. Eventuall,y I just hung up in anger. I called my mom, got in an argument with her too, and eventually hung up angry and pissed. It was about 4:30 in the afternoon and I had planned to go to a support group at 5:30. As I started driving to the meeting, a couple of crazy ideas came into my head. The first one was that I needed a smoke. I had not had a cigarette in a long time. On the corner was a small store where I stopped and bought a pack of Camel cigarettes. As soon as I lit up, I felt immediate relief. Ahh ... nothing like a good smoke. Then, as I was headed to group, I thought that I would stop at a downtown bar and pay off an old bar tab that was several years old. Perhaps if I made these financial amends, everything would be better.

What I did when I arrived at the bar was have three drinks in ten minutes. Shit, I was drinking again. My first thought was to go to the support group anyway, that nobody would know. But I didn't listen to that thought. Instead I thought what the hell, why not drink? So off I went into the night going from bar to bar.

Except for the beginning and the end, there is very little of that night that I remember. Blacked out—alcohol induced amnesia—again. Eventually I found myself back at my little apartment. The last thing that I drank was a bottle of cooking sherry that I had at home in my kitchen. I would never recommend drinking cooking sherry, but it was all I had. It was four in the morning on the 13th of December.

By ten in the morning my phone was ringing over and over again and my pager was buzzing. Two people were calling.

One was the sometimes girlfriend, the other was my boss. The woman ended up coming to my apartment and left angry. Shortly thereafter, my boss showed up. He knew that I had been working on being sober. He now saw me wiped out and hungover. My boss, possibly a drunk himself, went into action. First he said that he needed to get me to the hospital, that I needed help. Second, he told me that he would make sure that the stores I was responsible for were taken care of, that he would do it himself while I recovered in the hospital. Really, he would do that?

For the next six days I was at the hospital rehab, detoxing. The first few days, I was pretty much in bed, sick as a dog. I had consumed so much alcohol during my relapse, they told me, that I had alcohol poisoning. The image in SICU in 1971 of the dying alcoholic popped into my mind. *Fuck, was I now the dying drunk with the messed up liver?*

The time in the hospital rehab was rough. Hard doses of reality began to hit me. I truly was hopeless. Once I had the first drink there was nothing that I could do to stop. I was totally 100% powerless. I couldn't stop drinking any more than I can stop the rain. My initial sobriety had been built on quicksand. I had tried to use the woman to keep me sober. That didn't work. It was practically inevitable that the way I had been living my life, I would drink again.

CHAPTER 8

ON MY KNEES

Once I got out of hospital, I returned to the support groups with my tail between my legs. I had relapsed and had to admit it to my friends. Mostly, though, that was ok. Talking to another drunk is often what helps keep another drunk sober. One friend approached me and asked if I was done with drinking. I was so done and I knew it. This time I didn't swear off alcohol. The desire to drink had simply lifted. *My last drink was that cooking sherry on December 13, 1988. My first day of sobriety is December 14, 1988. With the grace of God I haven't had a drink since—nor will I ever have another drink again.*

One of my friends became a confidante that I could tell anything to. I told him everything that was going on in my life and my deepest darkest secrets. Confession of our mistakes and defects is a long-held spiritual principle. By sharing with another human being, God could remove those defects. Oh boy, did I have a lot of defects. In recovery circles it is said that you are only as sick as your secrets. I was pretty sick and it was time to get better.

For the next three months, my friend put me on an immediate and true course of action. Each week I was given something new to do. He had me start by really looking at my powerlessness over alcohol. That part had finally become easy. I then moved on to learning about the insanity of my disease, and that turning my will over to God would change that. The realization came to me that if I sought God, I would stay sober.

Next, my friend focused on helping me see my defects and where I had made mistakes. As we continued, I learned how to turn all this over to my higher power. One of the toughest parts was making a list of all those people I had harmed. It was difficult to see this, though slowly much of it came to light. The part I couldn't do anything about were all those times I had blacked out. Not much I could list there. I also had to go back to these people I had harmed to make amends. Sometimes people would take that well; other times, not so well.

Once my friend had gotten me through this maze of my life, he had me spend time in prayer and meditation. I really connected to the idea that taking time to just sit still would calm my mind. Often I would be on my knees asking for help and guidance. I was told to throw my shoes under my bed so I had to get on my knees to get them out. To complete the course of action, I was taught how helping another drunk was a key principle in creating the foundation to a sober life. To this day, whenever another drunk asks for help, I am there. Not only for them, also for me.

During this time, I was attending my support groups on a daily basis. I became quite active in helping out wherever I could. Sometimes I would set up chairs; other times I would clean ashtrays. Whatever I could do, I was happy to do it. Learning to become humble was something that I was striving for.

In addition to the regular support groups, I was part of a circle of men that had an interest in Native American practices. I didn't know much about that. Some of the men in the group were sober, the rest were not, and didn't need to be. We started out burning sage and smudging ourselves. This is intended as a cleansing process. Drumming was next. That I could get into. Once the drumming session was over, each of us would have an opportunity to talk. Each person who talked would hold the talking stick that was passed from person to person. This meant that no one could be interrupted when talking. I liked the no interruption part.

That group lasted about seven years. Being part of this group was really great for me. My relationship with my father went through many ups and downs, and I had been afraid to open up and get emotionally close to men. Learning to connect and talk to men had been difficult in much of my life.

The days of being sober turned into months. The months turned into years. Slowly my life was rebuilding on a new foundation. I had a good job and started meeting women that I liked. My father had passed away, but my relationship with my mother got much better. So did my relationships with the rest of my family and friends. My mind was clearing and a new relationship with God was developing, though I still didn't totally trust Him. That would take a while longer. Even with that, life was much, much better.

MOM HAS CANCER

November 1991, a month before my third year of sobriety, my mom was diagnosed with cancer. For about a year, she knew something was wrong in her body. She went to the doctor a number of times without any type of diagnosis. Mom had been at her home in Palm Desert playing golf, playing bridge and spending time with her many friends. Then, one day she was feeling so bad a friend took her to the hospital. It was at The Desert Hospital that they found the cancer. The tumor had grown to the size of a large grapefruit. Stage IV ovarian cancer.

Mom called me crying and devastated. She was afraid that she would die there and not be with her family. Dad had died in their desert home in 1985. Mom did not want to die there too. The doctors at Desert Hospital wanted her to have surgery immediately. Instead, she made the decision to return to her Portland home and be near family. Within days of being back in Portland, she had her first surgery. They were able to remove most of the cancer, but not all of it. Chemotherapy and radiation followed. The long-term diagnosis was not good.

After numerous hospital visits, surgeries and more chemotherapy, mom passed away in the middle of the night. She did not want to die. Mom was only 66 and wanted to live. She had put on a good face and lived her life, regardless of having cancer. Mom was at home in Portland and was surrounded by family and friends during her final days. When she did pass, it was the middle of the night and it was calm, quiet and peaceful.

I don't know how it happened. Dad had passed on Mother's Day, May 12, 1985. Mom passed May 23rd, 1994 on dad's birthday. How does that happen? The month of May is frequently a time of personal grief for the passing of my parents.

CHAPTER 9

LEARNING TO TWIST

Walking was on the top of the list as part of my ongoing exercise program. Before and after Pritikin, I would often measure the distance I would walk by the distance between light posts at Mt. Tabor Park. I joined Gold's Gym and I would do the stairmaster and treadmill until exhausted. All this effort helped to keep building new collateral blood vessels in my legs. Lifting weights was important, and I would venture into the aerobics classes from time to time.

In the aerobics room, there were yoga classes that normally had about 10 people. Though still a little goofy, occasionally I found the yoga classes to be "relaxing." Most of the postures were very difficult for me, but I would just do what I could. Normally, the teacher would finish class with savasana, relaxation pose. Just lying on my back doing nothing felt good. This was my favorite posture!

DIANE WILSON

One day I found an ad in the paper about yoga classes from someone named Diane Wilson. For some reason, I found the ad interesting and showed up for her class in downtown Portland. Right away I knew that Diane would be a yoga teacher of mine for some time to come. For several years, I continued to go to Diane's yoga class, almost daily. I found her a little wacky and the studio was decorated in a way I thought was goofy. There were pictures of spiritual people in colored robes. They reminded me of the spirits in the garden from my coma. There were huge paper butterflies hanging from the high ceiling and she would burn incense. I never liked the incense much—too much smoke.

From time to time, Diane talked about a guy named Ernest Wood as one of her primary yoga teachers. I thought, "Who in the heck is this guy?" He looked like a 60-year old typical business man from the South. I found out that he was a direct disciple of Paramahansa Yogananda, a yoga guru from India. At the time I had no idea who either Ernest Wood or Paramahansa Yogananda was.

Sometimes I would get a little bored with yoga and would bounce between the gym and Diane's. Eventually, I hired a personal trainer to help me at Gold's. James was a student at the National College of Naturopathic Medicine, making money on the side as a personal trainer. The first thing he had me do was a cleansing diet for 21 days. I thought I was going to starve. It was mainly juice, water, broccoli and a little bit of protein powder (to this day I still don't know if it did any good!).

James would tell me that, even though I wasn't the strongest person at the gym, it was clear I had tremendous endurance and that I would never give up. He would tell me what to do. I did it, and almost always did just a little bit more. Often, at the end of my training sessions, I would go to the corner and do some yoga postures. Whenever I did this, people scattered. I think they thought I was a little weird.

When I practiced yoga, I mostly went to Diane's classes, though began to venture out and try other classes. In 1993, I showed up at Bikram's Yoga College of India in Portland. The school had recently opened and I heard that the room was hot as hell. For some crazy reason, they would turn up the heat to something like 105. That seemed pretty insane. I went once and I thought it was hot, sweaty and stupid. There must have been something wrong with exercising in that hot of a room. When I did class, all the students in the room were sweating puddles everywhere. There was barely any sweat on me. I was nearly dry and felt overheated. So I went back to the gym and to Diane's classes.

With all this yoga and walking, my legs had gotten somewhat better, but I still had persistent pain in my left leg. I would rarely talk about the pain to my friends. My self-esteem was so low I thought that people would not like me if I seemed to be weak and complaining. Just like after my accident in seventh grade, I didn't want to feel rejected. So I mostly I kept the pain a secret from people. Often my calf would be screaming and my left foot would go numb. There still was not complete adequate blood flow to my leg.

BERYL BENDER BIRCH

Growing up and in high school, I loved to ski and really missed not being able to hit the slopes because of my legs. Even before skiers were doing it, I would leave one ski at the bottom and ride up the lift and ski down on one ski. At the time I was skiing on

Atomic 205's—pretty long skis for today. I missed all the fun of skiing and I was anxious to get back to the mountain.

One day I made up my mind and I went to the Portland Outdoor Store to buy brand new skis. This was a huge turning point for me. I thought that my legs would never let me ski again. Not only did I buy a new pair of skis, but I saw a flier on the wall for an upcoming yoga workshop that was starting the very next day.

The flier announced that Thom and Beryl Bender Birch taught something called "power yoga" to the U.S.A. Ski Team. I thought perfect, I've got to meet these people! The workshop was being held at Holiday Johnson's Studio in Portland. When I called to register, Holiday answered. I had never met her before, but we seemed to hit it off on the phone right away. She told me that the workshop had been filled for weeks and that there was a very long waiting list. Then Holiday paused and said somebody had just dropped out a few moments earlier. She gave me the opening spot in front of others that were on the waiting list. To say the least, I was totally jazzed and excited to be able to go.

The next day I showed up and Tom and Beryl started talking about Ashtanga Yoga and Power Yoga. I did not know much about either type of yoga. They said the workshop was for those people who were just beginning to learn the Ashtanga tradition. I was quite impressed with how both of them explained everything. I'm not sure exactly what their age was, but Beryl was about 10-15 years older than Tom. She described a long history of yoga in her life.

Tom had been a world-class marathon runner, one of the top 50 in the world. He described how he found Ashtanga Yoga after a career-ending injury, and how he learned through yoga practice to heal himself and to run again. What I remember strongly is his description of how he learned to breathe in a different way. He talked about how he would be in the lead pack with three or four other runners, with just a couple miles left. The other runners were all huffing and puffing. But because of his breathing practice he would kick into gear and race out in front of them with ease. I thought that was pretty amazing. Maybe I can start to let go of some of my leg pain and change some of the ways that I do things—and become an awesome skier.

The first session of the workshop was new and different for me. We started off with that same Downward Dog posture I used to fall out of. I thought, "I can do this, Diane taught me that." But what was so different was that we didn't only do the Downward Dog. We would jump through our arms into various postures. By the end of that first day I was hooked. I knew that Ashtanga was for me.

Something happened to me that had never happened before. At the end of the first day, we lay down on our backs in savasana. As Beryl was softly leading us through a meditation, I began to cry. For the next fifteen minutes, I had tears running out of my eyes into the carpet. I felt like a surge of energy was going through my spine and my body. This was a new sensation and was something I'd never felt before.

When we were finished, Beryl asked us to talk about our experience that day in class. I described my new-found joy and I that I had all this energy flowing through me. She explained it as a "kundalini" experience, where energy is moving through your spine. Maybe, maybe not. I don't know. There were two more days left in the workshop, during which I continued to deepen my practice and learned more about this thing called Ashtanga Yoga.

It felt like I had found my yoga practice—the hot Bikram Yoga was out, Diane Wilson was out, Power Yoga and Ashtanga were in. There was just one problem. There really wasn't anyone that I was aware of that taught Ashtanga yoga in Portland at that time. So there was really nowhere to take class.

DAVID SWENSON

Beryl had mentioned an Ashtanga teacher named David Swenson. He was one of the early Ashtanga practitioners in this country, and one of the first American teachers. Not only that; he was having a two-week yoga workshop in Costa Rica. I immediately signed up.

We spent two weeks at Basque del Cabo Wilderness Lodge, on the southern coast of Costa Rica. We practiced Ashtanga two times a day—once in the morning and once in the evening. There's nothing like practicing yoga, watching the toucans flying by, the howler monkeys in the trees, and being uncertain whether a poisonous snake would slither by.

David really helped me deepen my yoga practice. Here was a guy in his 40s who had done nothing but Ashtanga yoga, whose body was cut like a professional athlete. I thought maybe someday I can look like that too. Instead of feeling embarrassed about my body, I might actually feel good about my scarred up body.

After returning to Portland, I met other people who also liked Ashtanga yoga. A small group of us started something we called the Portland Ashtanga Co-op. We rented a space at One With Heart, a martial arts studio on Hawthorne Boulevard, and ended up with about a dozen people in each yoga session. Each of us would trade off leading the class, sometimes playing a tape of David's. Eventually we moved our class to the Yoga Space on southeast Ankeny. As we did this, our classes grew and so did our abilities. Some of us would go off on our own trips and study with various senior Ashtanga teachers.

Having met Clifford Sweete at Tom and Beryl's, we invited him to do a workshop for us in Portland. He was also one of the early Ashtanga practitioners in this country. He told a story of how he and David had picked up Pattabi Jois at the airport on his early visits to the United States. Pattabi Jois is the guru of Ashtanga Yoga.

NISCHALA JOY DEVI

I don't know the first time I found out about Nischala. Nischala had helped Dr. Dean Ornish establish his early program for reversing heart disease. She also was instrumental in the formation of the Commonweal Cancer Program. Both of these programs have a strong yoga component.

Because of my father's heart attack and my vascular disease, I had a great deal of interest in how yoga could keep heart disease away in my life. I simply wanted to keep living. I studied with Nischala and attended a two week certification on Yoga of the Heart. This program is used with individuals that are dealing with heart disease. The training helped give me additional understanding of working in hospitals, and with individuals with heart ailments and other chronic health conditions.

ERICH SCHIFFMAN

Sometime in the mid-90's I met Erich at Powell's Book Store in Portland. He was on a tour for a book he had just written on yoga. Erich immediately impressed me with what he said and how he said it. Someone in the audience asked him what he thought about a vegetarian diet. Basically his response was, "Sounds good to me—people should eat any way they want." Right on Erich!

Over the years I have attended his classes in Los Angeles many times. At one point in the mid '90's I went through Erich's teacher training and learned a huge amount about running energy in the body. Today I continue to have a deep respect for Erich and what he continues to teach.

MORE LEG PAIN

Though I rarely wanted to mention it to anyone, I was still experiencing ongoing pain in my left leg. Then something else began to happen. My left shoulder would frequently hurt after vigorous Ashtanga yoga sessions. Many times I would need to ice the shoulder to help cool it down, reduce the swelling and remove the pain. Eventually I went to the Sports Medicine Clinic at Emanuel Hospital. They diagnosed me with bursitis and tendonitis. Several x-rays were taken about a month apart and showed how the bones in my left shoulder were separating and how the acromion process was beginning to move. No wonder I was experiencing so much pain. In hindsight, I don't know if I'd been practicing downward dog with incorrect alignment, or whether the nature of the posture itself had created the injury and pain in my shoulder.

I felt as if I was now at another turning point in life. I was really excited about yoga, and it made my body feel so good. Yet I couldn't do the Ashtanga without continuing to hurt my shoulder in class. In the back of my mind I remembered Bikram's Yoga and the hot room. I remembered that they didn't do the downward dog at Bikram's. Maybe if I did the hot room for a while I could later come back to Ashtanga.

CHAPTER 10

HOT & SWEATY

I couldn't believe I was at Bikram Yoga again. It was such a hot, sweaty, twisted, stinky place. But my left shoulder had been killing me and I just wanted the pain to go away. I was simply tired of so much physical pain throughout my life. I was tired of how my emotions were all tied up with the struggles to be healthy and out of pain. When I started at Bikram's, I had plenty of doubts whether my pain would ever go away. However, I was very determined and didn't like giving up.

Bikram Yoga class starts with a breathing exercise where you lift your elbows to the ceiling. When this exercise started, there was a sharp pain in my left shoulder. The teachers told me that, if I wanted to heal my shoulder, I needed to practice every day. Really, everyday? Wouldn't that make it worse? Ok, I will do it anyway. After a month of daily practice, the shoulder pain was virtually gone. I will say that again—the shoulder pain was gone! The teachers were right.

Then I noticed something else. It was 1997 and the pain that I'd been carrying in my legs since my surgeries in 1986 seemed to be a little less intense. *The thought occurred that if my shoulder pain went away and my leg pain was getting better, perhaps I could I truly live a life without any pain. It was a totally startling concept for me. A life without pain? After so many years and tears, I had resigned myself to ongoing physical pain for the rest of my life.*

With a near daily practice now at Bikram Yoga, I found out that Bikram himself was doing a three month teacher training in Los Angeles starting in just a few months. I thought, "Do I really want to go to this guy for help?" Rumors had it that he was tough and mean. This did not appeal much to me. However, Gilly, who owned the school where I was taking classes told me, "Oh don't worry about Bikram Just go and learn what you can."

Even with that said, I continued my search for a place to immerse myself in yoga. Releasing the pain became a top priority in my life. I called and asked many leading teachers in different traditions if they could help me with my health. Since many of my friends who went to India got sick there, I wanted to stay in the United States.

After many phone calls and discussions, I found myself writing and mailing a check for $4,000 to Bikram—the cost of the training. My interest wasn't to become a teacher. I just wanted to further study in an intense manner with a yoga master and heal my aching body.

TEACHER TRAINING

My first time at Bikram's school in Los Angeles was a few days before the training started. The school was right on the very busy corner of Wilshire and Robertson in Beverly Hills. There was a steep black metal stairway in the back parking lot leading to the second floor entrance to the school. What a strange place for a master's yoga studio. I was full of anticipation and my left leg was hurting pretty good. Slowly I made my way up the daunting stairs. Walking around the school and the locker rooms, I couldn't help thinking, "What have I gotten myself into? This place is dumpy. I'm spending all this money and this is the best they can come up with?" I had figured with all the Rolls Royces that Bikram owned, his school would be state of the art. Compared to India, I suppose it was.

The room where yoga was practiced was the stinkiest place I had ever smelled. Bikram joked that it smelled like 1,000 donkeys farting. No doubt. On the walls were pictures of Bikram and his wife, Rajashree. The pictures showed them in all sort of weird postures that I'd never seen before and had no idea what many of them were called.

I was a little scared to meet Bikram because of the things I'd heard about him. Then the first time I saw him in person, I found he was really just a small, Indian man, not physically imposing at all. When I introduced myself and mentioned the problem with my legs, he just shrugged and said nothing. That bothered me. I figured he would want to know all about was going on with my health and in my body. What I really wanted was special attention because of my surgeries and injuries. Bikram didn't give it to me.

Before I knew it, several weeks had passed and we were having yoga class two or three times a day. Instead of just 90 minutes, Bikram would teach for two hours or more. Between classes we would have posture clinic where we would study each posture much more in depth. The posture I hated the most was dandayamana janushirasana, also known as "standing head to knee pose." This was the posture where I felt the most intense pain in my left leg.

One particular day in posture clinic, I asked Bikram about this posture and the pain. The memory is vivid. He sat on the floor 10 feet in front of me; one woman was brushing his hair and another woman was rubbing his arms and back. I said, "How do I modify the posture to reduce the pain?" He looked right at me and said, "Don't change anything." I said, "You don't understand Bikram. My calf really hurts. Somehow I have to modify the posture so it doesn't hurt so much." Bikram replied in his Indian accent, *"I know Michael, don't worry about, forget about it, just do the yoga."* In my head I was thinking, "Fuck you dude, give me my $4,000 back and go back to India. I came here for you to heal me." I didn't say what I thought and sat behind him and the group of other student teachers. It was all that I could do to stay put and not leave.

THE RELEASE

When I first got to Los Angeles for the training, I had met Kim at Whole Foods. She worked there in health and beauty aids and did massage on the side. We connected and every week during training I would go to her for a relaxing massage.

During this particular massage session, a totally unexpected release occurred. Kim barely touched my left calf and I felt terrible pain. The tears started flowing down my face. It was one of those very tearful blow-your-snot-out-of-your-nose types of moments. All sorts of emotions and memories of my relationship with my father came up. The arguments, the drinking, everything. Kim just held my leg with loving energy and let me sob and talk. This lasted over 30 minutes and I knew I was letting go of something. But what really happened?

The next morning in the 9:00 a.m. class, something totally new and unexpected happened. When I picked up my right foot and balanced on my left leg, the pain in my calf was gone. Continuing the posture, I kicked my right leg straight out. Still no pain in my left calf. Next I brought my elbows down around my right leg and touched my head to the knee. Tears came to my eyes, there was no more pain. Bikram always said, "Pain kills the pain, poison kills the poison." Hmm, is that part of what was happening? Had I let go of my emotional pain the night before that released the physical pain?

Bikram would mention his teacher Bishnu Ghosh, would say that 100% of all disease comes from stress. Is that what I was experiencing? *Had I released emotional stress in my mind that relieved my vascular disease and the pain in my body? If the yoga masters are right, then that is exactly what happened.* My opinion of Bikram Yoga began to change. I now began to understand just a little more how yoga works.

THE DOCTORS

As training proceeded, we had the following physicians that are experts on yoga therapy instructing us. Dr. Anne Marie Benstrom is a doctor originally from Sweden and owner of "The Ashram" north of Los Angeles. Dr. Bhaumik is a laser physicist who came from India. He was instrumental in the development of laser surgery, and holds a dozen patents in the field of lasers. He would talk to us about yoga and the super consciousness. Dr. Das visited us from Calcutta and spoke in depth about many of the medical aspects of the application of yoga therapy. He holds a double Master's Degree from

Calcutta University in Allopathic and Alternative medicine, and has a Ph.D. in Yoga Therapy. Dr. Chauduri is Professor and Executive Chair of the Department of Obstetrics and Gynecology and Distinguished Professor of the Department of Molecular and Medical Pharmacology at UCLA. He received his M.D. from India and his Ph.D. from London University under the mentorship of a Nobel Laureate. Dr. Frank Trapani, from Walla Walla, Washington, came next. Dr. Trapani is a chiropractor and an expert in nutrition.

Emmy Cleaves, the most senior Bikram teacher, lectured us a number of times. One of her lectures that I remember vividly was her talk on pain. Here was this woman, at the time in her 70's, who had taught us a number of yoga classes so far. I was astonished that a woman at that age could practice yoga and look so damned good. Emmy is now one of my most admired teachers.

Ok, now I am listening. This is exactly what I wanted to study and to learn. Bikram, Rajashree and all the teachers showing us "how yoga works." What I was learning was more than I could have imagined. I was beginning to understand and see how the body and mind really work. How the relationship of our thoughts affect what is manifested in our body. I was learning the correct therapeutic application of yoga asana. I was learning how to heal my body and how to help others heal their body. I still didn't want to be a teacher—but eventually that would change.

TEACHER GRADUATION

Near the end of the training, I felt as if I was in the best shape of my life. My leg pain was gone. When I first entered training, I weighed 180 pounds. During those three intense months I was sure I was losing weight. But at the end, I was 181 pounds. My body had simply been reshaped and now looked quite toned. More important, my leg pain was gone.

For graduation, I was chosen as valedictorian and asked to speak as the representative of my fellow graduating teachers. Along with five other teachers I was asked to participate in a yoga demonstration during the ceremonies. Both of these were a true honor for me. A funny note: Bikram had told me to shave my armpits because he thought they were too hairy for the demonstration. I didn't want to do that, so I told him no and still did the demonstration.

Before graduation, Bikram asked me to write my speech and what I was going to say. I resisted, but he kept insisting, and I just told him that I would talk about my experience in teacher training and yoga. I never did write anything and told him that I was going to talk about how I was no longer in pain. Still, until I started talking, I didn't what I would say for sure.

During the graduation speech, I wore a dark suit and a red tie. Yep, even yogis dress in suits. Often in the day to day teacher training, I had taken a lot of photographs of everything that happened. So the first thing I did when I got up on stage to talk was take several photographs of the audience. Bikram and everyone were howling in laughter.

In my speech I talked about everyone in training and what we had learned. I said that I was not planning to teach classes, that I would just help other teachers open their studios. After all, I knew how to run a business and knew how to set up multiple locations. Being excited that my leg pain had disappeared, I demonstrated standing head to knee pose in my suit. This created more clapping and laughter. It has been a great honor that, out of perhaps 8,000 plus teachers Bikram has trained, I was, maybe, teacher 125 to receive a teaching certificate in this system of yoga.

RETURNING TO PORTLAND

Returning to Portland after graduation, Gilly asked if I wanted to teach a few classes a week at her school. Well, ok, but I only wanted to teach two or three classes a week. Little did I know as I began to teach how much I would like it, and how much the students seemed to like the way I taught.

The insight and feedback from Gilly and her other teachers continued to teach me valuable lessons about yoga. At one point I thought it would be great to have my own school, which really surprised me, because having a yoga school was normally the last thing on my mind.

Then, one day, another teacher from Portland and I talked about opening a school in partnership together. Open a yoga school? Now everything was changing and quickly. Initially it made sense to own a school together, mainly because it would give me freedom to travel and do other things. But I wasn't certain whether Portland was big enough for two Bikram studios. We talked to Gilly about that and we decided Portland could handle a second Bikram school.

At about the same time, my girlfriend Sue and I drove to Bend, Oregon, to look at the possibility of opening a studio there. As the process of opening a studio went on—finding the space, fumbling through the actual logistics and with Bikram's blessing—I ended up opening the school on my own in Portland. In 1999, that was perhaps the 25th Bikram school in the world to open.

Being a school owner became really exciting—this was actually happening. After all the construction and tenant improvements were done and everything that it took to open the doors, it was a tremendous relief. It seemed as if the hard part of opening was now done. Students started to come in and the classes quickly filled. Many students had all sorts of problems and health issues that were getting better after just a few classes.

As I gained more experience as a teacher and studio owner, I was traveling to Los Angeles up to ten times a year. I wanted to study as much as I could with Bikram, Rajashree, Emmy and all the other teachers and doctors. During the ongoing teacher trainings, I would assist Bikram training new teachers. So far I have taught at 28 teacher trainings. Bikram would ask me to lecture to the group of teacher trainees and talk a bit about my personal story, basically on how my body had healed through the yoga.

All of this teaching and working with Bikram gave me a deeper understanding of what my personal experience was with the yoga and the why and how my body was healing. I learned that, often times, in yoga, and especially in life, it is so easy to get stuck in our own shit. What I was really learning was to walk through the pain, and not stay stuck in it. The key word here is "through."

Going back to my studio in Portland, I would bring my growing revelations back to the classes I taught. There were so many students that began to experience their own personal healing that I lost track. In my studio I saw many students with back pain. Some had bulging or herniated discs and other conditions that created pain in the spine and back. There were (and are) times that, after just one class, the pain would be gone. One student had a diagnosis of colon cancer and surgery was recommended. She committed to herself that she would practice every day for 40 days. When it was time for her surgery, the doctors were unable to find any cancer. I've seen people with diabetes reduce their need for insulin in half. There are endless testimonials of students overcoming the worst conditions you can possibly imagine.

BEND STUDIO
In the fall of 2003, I came to Bend to help my new girlfriend open a studio. At first it was 100% her studio, and I was driving back and forth to my Portland school. It was my intention at the time to be in Bend, teach some classes, hike and write this book. Instead, I first bought half the studio from her, then bought the remaining portion later on. In the meantime, I had sold the Portland studio and was now living in Bend full time.

CONTINUING TO LEARN
From 2003 to the present I have been 100% focused on teaching in Bend, continuing to assist Bikram at the trainings, and learning more and more about how yoga works. I would frequently practice the advanced series in LA with Emmy whenever I could. The understanding and knowledge of the practice grew exponentially. There were many "ahha moments" that would flood into my consciousness. When the Bishnu Ghosh Hatha Yoga Championships started, I was one of the original judges. Through all of this, Bikram has helped me to see and understand the effects of yoga at a much deeper level.

Rajashree has always been instrumental in expanding my understanding of Bikram Yoga. Here was this beautiful woman from Kolkota, India. From 1979 to 1983 she was the five-time winner of the All India Yoga Championships. Bikram said that is why he married her. Early in life, her teacher became Dr. Das. Eventually Rajashree received several certifications in India and is an expert in the application of hatha yoga for chronic disease and disorders. She has frequently taught and lectured about the intricate relationship between the mind and the body, and the manifestation of health conditions in the body, and how to heal with the application of yoga asana.

Since that first yoga class in 1987 at the Pritikin Center, my whole view of yoga has shifted. The main reason that I initially started yoga was to help my body heal. I wanted relief from physical pain and I found that is one of the greatest gifts that yoga has to offer.

In India hatha yoga is often used to help heal the body, and in many hospitals the body is first heated prior to the therapeutic application of a yoga asana. Earlier in my practice, I thought putting my foot behind my head was important. Today "learning to still the fluctuations of the mind" and being healthy is what I practice the most. I've found that as my personal practice has deepened and as I've learned to be an expert teacher, that the two—teaching others and practicing—are intricately linked. On some level, whether I own a school or not, I will always be a teacher.

CHAPTER 11

WHAT I LEARNED

W hy have I told you all these deeply personal stories about my life and falling on my face? First, it has been tremendously healing for me to open up and talk about what really happened. That, somehow, through the tragedies of life I have kept getting up whenever I have fallen.

What was it that kept me alive after the water skiing accident? What was my experience of the spirits in the garden all about? Why did they tell me to get back to my body? How had I drunk so much without killing myself or someone else? What was it that helped me get and stay sober? How in the world have I kept my legs after vascular disease? As Dr. Campbell said way back in 1971, it wasn't he that saved me. Perhaps it was God, a power much greater than anyone. Other doctors and friends have told me the same thing. You know what? I believe them. I have literally put one foot in front of the other, one step at a time. It was then through great willingness and trust in the process that grace has come into my life. As the spirits told me in the coma, "You are not through with this life, it is time to go back." Since I am still here, I guess I'm not done yet. There is more, so read on.

THE MASK

There he was lying on the ground covered with blood, motionless. I was standing over his dead body knowing that I had viciously killed him. Before I knew it I was arrested, charged and convicted of this heinous crime of murder. After being found guilty and with a sinking feeling in my gut, they transported me in a green bus to serve the rest of my life at state penitentiary. Sitting on the bench about half way back on the right side of the prison bus I could see the driver and the guard. My wrists were handcuffed and I was smoking a Marlboro. Somehow I found the handcuffs were loose and I could get out of them easily. Whenever the guard looked at me, I made sure that the cuffs appeared to be on. Whenever he wasn't looking at me, I would take the cuffs off and feel a sense of freedom.

Arriving at the prison, I got off the bus and found I was walking through the administration area all alone. Once I realized where I was, I simply walked out the front door and down the street. No one was following me; I was getting away.

Walking for about a half a mile, I came across a restaurant and went in. On the ground floor was the dining room, on the second floor was a plastic surgeon. I was so hungry and sat down to eat. Looking up, I saw the warden at a round table with a group of prison officials. I better get out of here before anyone of them recognizes me.

Thinking I would change my appearance, I headed up the stairs to the surgeon. Once the doctor did his thing, I knew that I wouldn't be recognized and would be safe from capture. Before the doctor started the operation, I changed my mind and headed back out the front door. If only I could drain my bank accounts and head to Mexico, my life would be decent. It would be much better than rotting in prison the rest of my life.

There was a pay phone in front of me and I called my friend Gary. I told him what happened. How I had killed somehow. How I escaped and how I was headed south of the border. *Right then I realized I could not live my life always hiding from others and constantly on the run.*

Suddenly I woke up. It was all a dream—or was it? It seemed so vivid and real, so lucid. Lying there in my bed, I was shocked that my mind would create such a disturbing dream. Could I really have murdered somebody? Was I really capable of such an act? I'm thankful that I never had to find out.

Once I got over the shock, I began to reflect on the dream and wonder if there was some message or meaning behind it. Pulling out my bedside dream dictionaries, I looked up the symbols that had appeared in the dream. Symbols like the murder, handcuffs, the bus, the warden, the plastic surgeon and so on. My interpretation began to give me a great sense of relief. It was a dream of contradictions. Killing somebody had really been about killing and removing parts of me that I no longer needed. Parts that were holding me back in life. More realization developed that whenever other people were looking at me I was not being myself. But when they looked away, I felt a sense that I could just be myself. *It was time to stop running away from who I was, to begin to remove the mask that I was using to hide behind in my life. Essentially time to accept myself for who I am.*

This dream happened early in my sobriety. The memories of the dream are still as strong as the night it happened. The lesson that it gave me is a constant reminder to just be myself. Am I always myself? No, frequently I will hide behind my many masks. This is the place I go to when I don't want others to know what I am thinking and feeling. Sometimes that seems to be a safer and easier place to be. Today I no longer need to drink or hide behind the bottle. I have found a new way to live. I have found that I have a higher power that guides and nudges me on a daily basis.

To truly live a life with my head up, with a strong sense of self-esteem, and learning to be willing to be humble and learn from my mistakes, is not easy. After all, some mistakes I do repeat. Perhaps I just haven't learned that particular lesson yet. Frequently, using prayer, I ask for the ongoing willingness to have my many shortcomings removed. I'm not looking for perfection, just a sense that I am making progress. Some of my defects may have been removed, many others are well entrenched. Thus the prayers will continue.

LESSONS FROM MY PARENTS

The early lessons from parents were pretty straight up. In the morning, make your bed when you get up; then you can have breakfast. When you are done eating, put your silverware on the plate at 10:20. Wait for everyone to finish their food before getting up and clearing the table. Wash the dishes. Wash your own clothes. Open doors for others whenever possible, especially for women. When walking with a woman on a road, always protect her by walking on the outside. Use proper names when talking to others. Respect your elders.

My parents taught me that there would be many times in life that I would fall down. They would remind me that no matter how many times that happened, get back up and just keep on going. I was told that there would be times in life to watch out for bullies, that many even lived right in our neighborhood. Sometimes I found that out the hard way and got beat up. Eventually I learned to stand up for myself and others that were getting picked on. My parents told me that bullies existed throughout the world and that, as I made my way through life, these bullies would appear from time to time at unexpected moments and unexpected places. Not just the physical bullies, but the emotional and mental bullies as well. Many of those bullies would be hiding everywhere, as a friend or in business. That many of them would put you down for any reason at all and try to take what you have. My parents taught me that if a shark was swimming towards me, it was their nature to try and eat me. But it was my responsibility to swim away before I became lunch. They also taught me that sometimes you have to stand up for what is right.

Perhaps one of the biggest lessons that I learned from my mom was courage. I didn't always follow her example. I did watch her stand up for what she believed in. Especially after dad passed, mom struggled to find her way. There were times when other people did not think she was doing the best thing. Whether she was or not, I don't know. I do know that watching her play out what she thought was right took tremendous courage. When mom was diagnosed with cancer, she always tried to maintain a smile and live her life. During her last couple of years before passing, she would do everything she could to remain grateful for all that she had. To the end, she showed great courage in all she did.

Dad always said you have two ears and one mouth. Listen twice as much as you talk. He said if I learned that, people would say anything, because people don't like the silence. Laugh as much as you can. Go to ballgames and sing. We used to go to the Portland Beavers together, have hot dogs and cracker jacks, sing all the songs, and root for the home team. Work hard and save your money. This is a lesson I am still working on. Through many of the challenges I saw my father go through, at the end of the day his family was always most important.

HEALTH

Don't believe everything the doctors say. They don't know everything and are often at a loss to explain what is happening in the body. This means that you have to trust what you believe in. If a certain drug or procedure doesn't seem right, don't do it. I studied and become aware of my physical ailments that were affecting my life. I learned to appreciate that a healing process is often quite simple and costs little or no money. Never underestimate the power of simplicity in healing. Our body rarely is missing some unknown ingredient in prescriptions. More than anything, the body just needs to be returned to its natural order. If you are sick, unhealthy or injured, be willing to try alternatives. Remember to never give up before the miracle happens.

SOBRIETY & ADDICTIONS

How do I say this? Ok, I will be straight up. Virtually everyone has some sort of addiction present in their life. Whether that is a personal addiction or the effects of the addictions from family, friends and co-workers. Especially if you are personally dealing with substance abuse, be willing to get help. Willingness to step up and accept ourselves— the willingness to have the courage to face our faults—can and will help us to make the change to a better life. It is said that for an alcoholic or addict, resentments are the number one offender. Find a friend or someone that you can talk to on a personal level to get help. In virtually every community, there are many organizations where help is available at little or no cost.

YOGA

The yoga masters of the past and the present have offered much wisdom about healing our bodies and our minds. Perhaps one of the deepest lessons I have learned in yoga was from Bikram. "Don't worry about, forget about, just do the yoga." This apparently simple statement is packed with so much power. Many times in my life, I needed to learn to let go of the worry and stress I put on myself, and trust the process. With a busy day-to-day life, it can often feel, inside my mind, like a monkey is scratching to find a banana to eat. Sometimes I might have so much stress there is a whole troupe of monkeys fighting over one little yellow banana

One of the first premises of yoga is "learning to still the fluctuations of the mind." Properly applied, the therapeutic benefits of yoga asana can help calm this chatter and give us stillness. This feeling of calmness will begin to radiate throughout our body and life and help give us deeper appreciation for ourselves and everything around us.

THE GARDEN

When I first experienced "The Garden" in my coma, I didn't want to come back to my body. I wanted to stay with the spirits. The Garden was a place that was free of pain. When I did return to this body, I developed a huge sense of abandonment. Abandonment from God and the spirits, and abandonment from my parents. I'm not saying they abandoned me. I'm saying that is what I felt and thought. I fought and struggled with this for years and experienced overwhelming resentment. This initial tiny seed of resentment grew quickly into anger, fear and self-pity. These feelings fed my underlying drinking and substance abuse. Eventually, my body was beginning to die and the doctors were ready to amputate me one leg at a time. Something happened though. I wanted to live.

To be able to live, my life needed to change. First, I had to admit that I was not in charge and be willing to turn my life over to the higher power that I was most angry with. Once I was able to do that, my higher power guided me to people and experiences that could help me. Slowly, I was taught how and where these seeds of anger and resentment were growing, and I was shown how to remove those weeds from my life. When those weeds were removed, the seeds of peace and love could flourish with the proper nourishment.

Learning to weed "The Garden" is what has kept me alive and what I continue to do today—one day at a time. I have discovered that I don't need to leave my body to feel peace. One day I know I will leave, though I can't tell you when. In the meantime, I know that "The Garden" is everywhere—it's learning to find the beauty of the path. As my journey continues and as I fall down from time to time, I hope that I have the courage to always get back up.

FINDING YOUR
OWN JOURNEY

Each of us needs to find our own way and must decide for ourselves what is right. If you are struggling with anything in your life, perhaps ask yourself the following questions:

- Do I want to keep struggling with this or am I ready to release it?
- Do I have a health condition that I want to heal?
- Do I have an addiction that is affecting my life?
- Is my life what I want it to be?
- Am I willing to do whatever it takes to feel happy, joyous and free?

Now, take an honest look at your answers. If you don't like what you see, make a decision now to do something about it. Don't wait until tomorrow. If you wait, the change may never come. Remember the Chinese proverb: "A journey of a thousand miles starts with a single step." With that in mind, what can you do now to begin your journey to something new in your life? Start with a simple plan of action. Read through the following ideas and start your own "Getting Up Project."

HOLD YOURSELF ACCOUNTABLE WITH ANOTHER PERSON

Talk to your partner or a friend and ask them to help you. Check in with them on a daily basis—even for a minute or two—and let them know what you are doing that day to make your life more fulfilling. If you are attending yoga classes, challenge yourself to 30 days in a row.

TAKING CHARGE OF YOUR PHYSICAL HEALTH

If you have any serious health problems, be sure to seek medical attention before you start. This is a good way to measure your progress. What are your vitals such as blood pressure, heart rate, cholesterol, weight, height and so on? Record what you can do each week to watch your changes. The only comparison you should make is with yourself—never anyone else.

Following are suggestions that anyone in any condition can do. If you find yourself in a hospital bed, start with a deep breathing exercise. Often there is a lot of stale air in our lungs that just needs to be replaced with fresh oxygenated air. Perhaps do focused breathing every hour—you just might surprise yourself and the medical staff.

Perhaps you are someone who is relatively healthy, and you just need a nudge to get started on taking better care of yourself. Start moving your body today. Begin with walking and yoga. Maybe walk to your local yoga studio. The combination of the two will restore your health quicker than you can imagine.

EASY START — FIRST PHASE

1. **Breathe.** Close your eyes and take three slow easy breaths. In through the nose, out through the mouth. This will calm the mind, reduce effects of stress and balance the central nervous system. This will increase oxygen in the blood and change the biochemistry of the body.
2. **Stretch the body.** Stretching. From a standing position, stretch right, left, back & forward. This gets the blood moving, affects the skeletal system and your internal organs. It is good for the health of your whole body.
3. **Walk.** Take a simple 10 minute walk around the block. A half-mile walk is approximately 1,000 steps. Five miles is approximately 10,000 steps. Walking is known to lower LDL (bad cholesterol) and raise HDL (good cholesterol); this helps to increase the health of the heart. You can Google "benefits of walking" to find many more benefits.

NEXT STEP — PHASE 2

1. **Yoga.** Yoga is the perfect foundation for all your other activities. Yoga helps to maintain, heal and strengthen the whole body and mind. Find the closest studio and sign up for a year of class. You will find yourself a brand new person and it will make everything else in your life that much better.
2. **Bike.** Start biking to work or just for fun. It is great for the legs and the lungs and saves a lot of gas.

3. **Swim.** Swimming is good for all your muscles and is great for rehabilitation.

CHALLENGE YOURSELF - PHASE 3

1. **Local Race.** Commit to a local marathon, triathlon or charity walk. Find something you like and grab a friend to train and complete the event.
2. **Kayak, Climb, Ski.** Try something you have always wanted to do, but have never done. Sign up for lessons and meet new friends.
3. **3 Hours Each Month to Charity.** Giving time to help others can be one of the greatest joys in life. Perhaps you give time to a soup kitchen, a pediatric ward in a hospital, or help a charity. Or even something as simple as making a large thermos of coffee on a cold winter day and giving free coffee to the homeless.

Taking Charge of Your Mental Health

Physical, mental and spiritual health go together. Just beginning to move your body will help you feel better about yourself. Science has shown that exercise helps to reduce depression. If you struggle with addictions, get proper professional care and find support groups.

EASY START – PHASE 1

1. **Make a list of what you want to change in your life.** Writing what you want to change makes it real.
2. **Make a gratitude list of everything you are thankful for.** Sit down and think of as many things as you can that you are thankful for. It might start simple—like the couch you are sitting on. Then look at work, family,

friends and people around you. On a daily basis, write down a minimum of five things you are grateful for. You just might surprise yourself.

3. **Talk to a friend about what you are doing.** This is one of the most important things you can do. Verbalizing and talking to a friend can help you speak what you want to change. The more personal you can be the better. It is said that we are only as sick as our secrets.

NEXT STEPS – PHASE 2

1. **Learn meditation.** Traditionally, most people think of meditation as sitting in lotus pose with your eyes closed. Perhaps you might want to learn that way. The easiest way to start is to simply sit upright in a chair, close your eyes and count 10 breaths. This alone can help your mind become more still. Deepen your practice anyway you want.

2. **Join a spiritual community.** Being around like- minded people is excellent for the soul. Ask friends and family for recommendations. Try different places. You might find strong connections in multiple places.

3. **Help someone else.** Helping someone else helps us get us out of ourselves. When we listen to a friend or help at a local charity, we are giving our time to something that helps everyone. This could be as simple as helping your neighbor.

GOING DEEPER – PHASE 3

1. **Go on a personal retreat.** When was the last time you took three days to yourself? Just went to the coast, rented a room, read a new book and walked the beach.

Maybe it is something more. Find a meditation retreat or something that appeals to you and just spend some quiet time with yourself.

2. **Join a support group.** This is especially important if you have any health issues such as cancer or addictions. Finding and talking to someone in your same situation can reassure us that we are not alone.

3. **Talk to a coach or a counselor.** Are you working through something that might be helped by working with a professional? If you know friends that work with coaches or counselors, ask them for a recommendation. Perhaps talk to several professionals on the phone to see if they might be right for you. Ask them if they work with your particular situation.

The whole idea about Finding Your Own Journey is to begin living a truly amazing life. It is easy to react to that which happens to us. It takes courage to step up and follow our inner guidance to live a life that we were meant to live. When we are able to follow that guidance, life just seems to fall into place with much greater ease.

RESOURCES FOR YOUR JOURNEY

"THE GETTING UP PROJECT"
"Providing ideas and resources to help individuals live a life with passion."

Everyone I have ever met has a story about their life to tell. Some are able to tell it with ease, others need encouragement to be able to let the story out. Often, our greatest success in life comes from our greatest challenges and failures. Once our stories are told, a new power can emerge from both the teller and the listener. The teller's power can come from just sharing their story, whether by pen or by mouth. The listener's power can come from reading or hearing the story, and relating to what they hear. This is the foundation of GUP. People relating to people.

What we do at "The Getting Up Project"

1. Offer a platform for individuals and businesses to create their stories of challenges and success.
2. Offer a platform to use your life as a way to take action, to move forward.
3. Offer ideas and resources to experience deeper passion and success in life.

To Start Action on Your Own
"Getting Up Project"
Visit the Website Now:
www.TheGettingUpProject.com

A Few Helpful Websites

Michael Harris
You will find more information about Michael Harris at the following websites, including additional books, upcoming trainings, workshops and media events. www.michaelbharris.com, www.fallingdowngettingup.com and www.thegettingupproject.com

Bikram Yoga
For information about Bikram Yoga, and to find a studio near you: www.bikramyoga.com

Meditation
For information about Holosync and learning to meditate. www.centerpointe.com

Heart Attack Proof
For information about preventing and reversing heart disease:
www.heartattackproof.com

Almine Barton, Lac, C.F.T.
An amazing blog about living life to its fullest. www.
alminewellness.blogspot.com

Addictions
If you are struggling with addictions in your life or those around
you, be sure to find local organizations that can help. Following
is the Wikipedia site that lists many groups specializing in
helping those with addictions. www.en.wikipedia.org/wiki/
List_of_twelve-step_groups

A FEW HELPFUL BOOKS

"How to Win Friends & Influence People"
by Dale Carnegie

"The Starfish and the Spider"
by Ori Brafman & Rod A. Beckstrom

Bikram Yoga
by Bikram Choudhury

How Yoga Works
by Genshe Michael Roach and Christie McNally

Prevent and Reverse Heart Disease
by Dr. Caldwell Esselstyn

The Biology of Belief
by Dr. Bruce Lipton

Divided Mind
by Dr. John Sarno

Surf is Where You Find It
by Gerry Lopez

Oh, The Places You'll Go
by Dr. Seuss

SUBMITTING YOUR STORY

So far in this book, I have written about myself—what happened and how I got through all the chaos. What I really want to know now is how you did it. Many people, really everyone—probably you—have incredible stories of Falling Down Getting Up. What is your compelling personal story? Would you like to have your story included and published in a future collection of similar stories in an upcoming book? If your story is selected for publication within a future printed book or e-book, we will pay you $200 and provide you with five printed copies of the book. Following are simple guidelines to submit your personal story.

1. The story must be a personal story about how you have been able to get back up after falling down. The story could be about just about anything that you have done

to stand up one more time. Perhaps you have experienced and overcome health, addiction, financial or relationship challenges. Virtually anything you have experienced is acceptable. All stories must be yours, real and non-fiction.

2. Please keep your story to between 750 and 1,500 words. Be specific and descriptive of what happened and what you were/are feeling. It is best if you can write directly from your experience in the first person.

3. All stories must be submitted by email. Preferred format is to write your story in Word or in the body of your email. You will receive an email confirmation upon your submission. We are not able to receive stories by regular mail or by fax.

4. You must include your full name, contact information and an active email with your submission.

5. If your story is chosen for publication and you wish for your name to remain anonymous, please let us know when submitting your story. For example, instead of using the name Steve Jones, we can label the author of a published story Steve J.

6. Keep a copy of your story. Due to the volume of stories we receive, it is impossible to send you copies.

7. Your story could be selected for publication in various formats including on-line, print or electronic. You agree that your story could be edited for such publications and used in different formats.

8. If your story has been selected for publication, we will notify you by email and request permission from you to use. We will not print anything without final permission

from you. If we are unable to contact you, we will not publish your story.

9. It often takes months or several years to publish personal stories. Please be patient and know that all stories may not be selected.

Please submit your story now to
www.thegettingupproject.com

EPILOGUE

The intention in writing this book has been two-fold: first, to write down what my experience has been; second, to show you and others that there is hope in life. That no matter how far you or I have fallen, that no matter how deep the hole is, that there is a way out. That it is never too late to start over. That if I can do it, you can too.

The stories I have told about falling down are very personal. Some friends and people who know me will be surprised at the depth of my struggles and the candor of my words. I am somewhat surprised, too, at my openness. Though I have never been interested in public office, that door is certainly closed now.

Then there are many stories of my life that I have simply not included in this book. There was the time I found myself face down in the gutter in the middle of a rainy night as I struggled to walk home after a night of drinking. I woke up later in bed with an open wound on my chin that required 10 stitches. There were many times as teenagers that a group of us would head for the Coast range of Oregon in our trucks filled with beer and pot.

There were also many more stories of success and gratitude. In the early 90's I had a job as an assistant controller of a business and learned much about accounting and banking. This helped me learn about the underlying functions of business. Later, I worked with a number of financiers on multi-million dollar projects that included everything from a music studio to luxury hotel projects. This helped me to see many business ventures in new ways.

Today I find myself in new transitions that are occurring in my life. That includes a new passion for writing, speaking and helping others on different levels. My movement from a business owner in these new directions is exciting and carries some uncertainty. Yes I have my goals and intentions, yet I know that, sometimes, the best laid plans get changed along the way. As more books are written and more talks are given, there will be times that I fall down, though I now know that that is part of the deal—as long as I get back up. For the day I don't get back up is the day that I just might die.

Start Your Own
"Getting Up Project"
www.TheGettingUpProject.com